Fix your eyes on the greatness of endoscopy as you have it before you day by day, fall in love with the subject, and when you feel it great, remember that this greatness was won by men with courage, with knowledge of their duty, and with a sense of honor in their deeds... So they gave their minds and bodies to the Society and received, each for his own memory, praise that will never die, and with it the grandest of all sepulchers, not that in which their mortal bodies are laid, but a home in the minds of men, where their achievements remain fresh to stir speech or action as the occasion comes by. For the whole Earth is the sepulcher of famous men; and their story is not graven only on stone over their native earth, but lives on faraway, without visible symbol, woven into the stuff of other men's lives. For you now it remains to rival what they have done and, noting the secret of happiness to be knowledge and the secret of knowledge an inquiring mind, not to idly stand aside from the eternal quest to heal.

Adapted from Thucydides (c. 460-400 B.C.)
The Funeral Oration of Pericles

I acknowledge that no man has a right to dedicate to others what is not his to own, particularly the past. Thus it is with this brief history of those who pursued the inner view. All that is mine in this modest little book is its recondite infelicities. These I dedicate to oblivion and with still avid yearning to the cerulean skies (*blou van onse hemel*) and the distant lonely reaches (*die ver verlate vlakte*) of the burning Karoo (*Une Saison en Enfer*). The rest belongs entirely to two extraordinary mentors, Barbara and Morton. Their exquisite and often diaphanous wisdom unveiled images for me in the dark mirrors of time and divulged the understanding that the mind's eye is infinite in both its scope and perception. Although I recognize that no oblation could adequately recompense so wondrous a gift, I dream that this *opus* may in some small part attest to my gratitude.

"As pines
Keep the shape of the wind
Even when the wind has fled and is no longer there
So words
Guard the shape of Man
Even when Man has fled and is no longer there."

Giorgios Seferiades (1900-1971)
"On Stage" 1966

Irvin M. Modlin, M.D., Ph.D., FRCS (Ed), FRCS (Eng), FCS (SA), FACS
Professor of Surgery
Dir., Gastric Surgical Pathobiology Research Group
Yale University School of Medicine
Department of Surgery
P.O. Box 208062
New Haven, Connecticut 06520-8062
USA

Editorial Director: Prof. Irvin M. Modlin

Associate Editor: Charles Lightdate

Art direction: Bruno Stucchi, Milano

Editing and coordination: Cicero, Milano

Illustration Design and Configuration: Irvin M. Modlin

Illustration Composition: M. Battaglin, J. Fahardi, M. Kidd, L.H. Tang

Typesetting and layout: Design Oltre, Milano

Separations and lithography: Fotolito Farini, Milano

Printed by Arti Grafiche Pizzi, Milano

Published by MultiMed, Milano

IRVIN M. MODLIN

A BRIEf
HISTORy
Of
ENDOSCOPy

ACKNOWLEDGEMENTS

IV

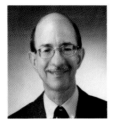

Charles Lightdale

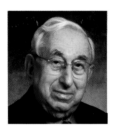

Joseph Kirsner

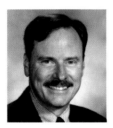

Jim Edmonson

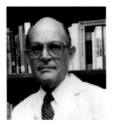

Basil Hirschowitz

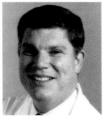

Lawrence Friedman

I am particularly indebted to Jim Frakes without whose foresight, friendship and support this work would never have seen the light of day. In addition, I recognize that without the perspicacity of the Governing Board of the ASGE who provided the means whereby I could view the past no such text would have been possible. I am grateful for the opportunity they have afforded me to allow the membership of the society, of which I am privileged to be a member, to share their vision that the road to the future is indeed an extension of the past.

A number of individuals provided me with wonderful insight to the world of vision and its visceral perspectives. Their time, advice and support contributed immensely to the pleasure of my task. Charlie and Reena Lightdale were not only extraordinarily patient with my ignorance of endoscopy and limited understanding of Burgundian benefice, but delightfully guided me through the flexible interstices of the American language. The proof of the vintage of their contributions may be found in every word of this text. As the sole survivor of the original founding meeting of the Society in 1941, Joseph Kirsner provided me with a rare view into history and the people behind the lens. Transfixed by his legendary maieutic skills I warrant that the Quadrangle has rarely witnessed a longer lunch and a more avid listener than I. Basil Hirschowitz with inimitable style and panache provided me with a unique perspective of the malleable nature of progress and illuminated for me the arcana of optics. William Haubrich, a gentleman and scholar, provided wisdom and an overview of the warp and woof of the history of the society. Larry Friedman was generous in overlooking my institutional affiliation and provided me with valuable insights as to the society and especially the role of "Blind Bennie". I owe a great debt of gratitude to Jim Edmonson (*Il miglior fabbro**), curator of the archives of the society and a scholar of rare wisdom and intellectual generosity. A perusal of his texts is to see the past as if it were today.

The amalgam of the sagacious contributions of my friends and colleagues as well as the most generous support provided by an unrestricted educational grant from Astra Zeneca LP, the Olympus Optical Co Ltd. and Olympus America Inc. facilitated the consummation of this felicitous endeavor. In this respect I am especially grateful to Tom McCourt of Astra Zeneca for helping to swiftly alleviate the dyspepsia and retrosternal discomfort that accompanies excessive verbosity. I am similarly indebted to Hiroshi Ichikawa of Olympus, whose cryptomeriad skills provided me with valuable endoscopic as well as gastronomic insight as he patiently educated me as to the differences between *unagi* and endoscopes.

Tiziana Paglia, Michele Buzzi and Bruno Stucchi of Milan deserve the highest commendation not only for their rigorous criticism and creative design, but the equanimity with which they bore my obsession with detail and esoterica. They accepted without complaint and with fortitude my refusal to accede to their request that the book be entitled either "*From Bozzini to Brunello*" or "*Visions of Amarone*". Without their substantial skills this risotto-like melange of history and clinical science would never have crystallized into a perceivable form. Irrespective of any possible refutations pursuant upon the time constraints afforded me, I am entirely responsible for any errors, oversights and misinterpretations of either history or scientific data expressed in this text.

I am especially obliged to a number of friends and colleagues. J. Fahardi and M. Kidd, of my research group for their amaranthine contributions to my current obsession. M. Battaglin and L. Tang who provided support in helping assemble and design the pictures that so facilitated the work of Bruno Stucchi and his Milanese colleagues. Shelley Robinson who nobly endured my slurred Capetonian accent and transcribed this text with exquisite patience, skill and good humor. George Sachs, whose understanding of the world of imagery and sagacious musing over the intellectual legacy of the Austro Hungarian Empire fructified the seeds of this endeavor. In his self anointed capacity as *Atropis* he adumbrated against the perils of excessive vision and abjured me from proton overload and rebarbative comment regarding "*matters gastrique or les estomacs.*"

My greatest debt is to Yale University School of Medicine and in particular the History of Medicine Library that provided me with the ideal milieu to pursue these studies. The archives of the ASGE proved to be a rich source of material and with the permission of the Society I have with gratitude mined deeply. Numerous institutions and individuals generously provided me access to material and allowed its usage. These include the *Yale University History of Medicine Library; the Huntarian*

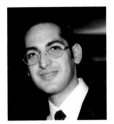

Jian Fahardi

Museum and Library of the Royal College of Surgeons of England; the Royal Society of Medicine; the Royal College of Physicians of England; and the Wellcome Institute for the History of Medicine. Institution; Blackett Laboratory, Imperial College of Science, Technology and Science, London; Blass Communications, Old Chatham, N.Y.; Broadmoor Hotel, Colorado Springs, CO; Chicago Medical School. Public Relations, Chicago; Cleveland Clinic, Public Relations, Cleveland, Ohio; Francis A.. Countway Library of Medicine, Boston, Mass; George Washington School of Medicine, Washington DC; Lenox Hill Hospital, New York; Olympus Optical Co. Ltd.; Moss Tubes, Inc., W. Sand Lake, N.Y.; New York Academy of Medicine, Historical Collections, New York; Rockford Gastroenterology Associates, Ltd., Rockford; University of Bern, Historical Library of Medicine, Bern; University of Cincinnati, Medical Center Academic Information Technology and Libraries, Cincinnati, Ohio; Windermere Hotel, Chicago.

Personal material was kindly provided by innumerable colleagues, scientific collaborators, and friends who have generously allowed me to use information emanating from their work or personal collections; *Ars Gratia Artis.* These include: *Dorothy Benson, Royal College of Surgeons in Ireland, Dublin, Ireland; Rebecca R. Bonsaint, ASGE, Manchester, MA; Brad Byers, Sword swallower, Moscow, Idaho; Tina Craig of the Royal College of Surgeons Library, London; James Edmonson, Cleveland Medical Library Association; Dittrick Medical History Center of Case Western Reserve University Ohio; Jian Fahardi, Yale University; Lawrence S. Friedman, Massachusetts General Hospital, Boston, MA; Martin E. Gordon, Yale University, New Haven, CT; William S.H. Aubrich, La Jolla; Hideki Mitooka, Kobe Seasde Hospital, Japan; Basil Hirschowitz, University of Alabama, Birmingham; Bernie C. Kern, Denver, Colorado; Mark Kidd, Yale University; Joseph B. Kirsner, University of Chicago Hospitals, Chicago, Carol Kirtz, Waban, Massachusetts; Lightdale Charles J., Columbia Presbyterian Medical Center, New York; Philip A. LoPresti, Jamaica Hospital, Jamaica; Machado Glaciomar, Rio de Janeiro, Brazil; Norman Marcon, R..S. DaCosta., Wilson B.C., Wellesley Central Hospital, Toronto; John W. Martin, Cameron-Miller, Inc., Chicago,Ill; John Morrissey, Bend Oregon; Jeffry L. Ponsky, The Cleveland Clinic Foundation, Cleveland OH; Hans J. Reuter, Max-Nitze-Museum, Stuttgart, Germany; Bernard M. Schuman; Medical College of Georgia, Augusta; Nicholas Wright Prof, Imperial College of Science, Technology and Science, London.*

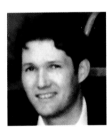

Mark Kidd

I wish to especially acknowledge the memory of two men whose magnificent achievements have for the most part been overlooked in the flow of time. In 1841 Daniel Colladon of the University of Geneva was the first to demonstrate light guiding and conceive that it could be bent around corners. Although his invention of compressed air powered devices eclipsed his optical studies, it was the latter principles which when applied to the fountains of Paris earned it the sobriquet of "The City of Light" and provided the basis whereby future scientists understood that light could be "piped".

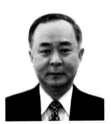

Hiroshi Ichikawa

Heinrich Lamm, while a medical student in Munich in 1930, attended the demonstrations of Schindler and recognized that the future lay in bending the light not the instrument. His novel experiments with glass fibers and the successful transmission of an image failed to achieve the recognition they warranted and his accurate prediction that such technology would result in the construction of a flexible gastroscope was lost in the chaos surrounding his eviction from Nazi Germany.

Lastly all whom have ever passed an endoscope owe an eternal debt of gratitude to the peripatetic genius of Rudolf Schindler (*qui genus "endoscipio" ingenio superavit***), whose perspicacity, tenacity and vision allowed him to not only see farther, but in so doing empowered us to share his vision.

Ave atque vale.

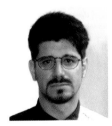

Bruno Stucchi

* The better workman. T.S. Elliot to Ezra Pound, *"The Waste Land"*.

** *He surpassed the race of endoscopists in understanding. (Apologia Newton)*

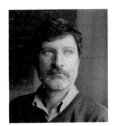

Michele Buzzi

Contents

Section I | *Overview of the Origins of Gastroenterology*   I

Chapter 1 | A Brief History of Gastroenterology   2

Chapter 2 | The Development of the Stomach Tube   10
EMPTYING THE STOMACH   10
INSTRUMENTATION OF THE STOMACH   11
THE STOMACH BRUSH   12
AN ESOPHAGEAL APPLICATION   14
ARTIFICIAL FEEDING   14
TREATMENT OF POISONING   16
THE CONTRIBUTIONS OF KUSSMAUL   19
DIAGNOSTIC USAGE   20
DUODENAL EVALUATION   22

Section II | *The Evolution of Diagnostic Instruments*   25

Chapter 1 | Bozzini and the Bladder   26
INTRODUCTION   26
UROLOGICAL ENDOSCOPY   26
PHILIP BOZZINI OF FRANKFURT   27
PIERRE SEGALAS (1792–1875) OF PARIS   28
JOHN FISHER (1797–1850) OF BOSTON   29
ANTONIN J. DESORMEAUX (1815–1881) OF PARIS   29
FRANCIS CRUISE (1834–1912) OF DUBLIN   31
MAX NITZE - A WORKABLE CYSTOSCOPE   33

Chapter 2 | Gastrointestinal Endoscopy   35
OPEN TUBES AND SWORD SWALLOWERS   35
OPTICAL SYSTEMS AND TUBES   36
ESOPHAGOSCOPY AND JOHANN VON MIKULICZ   37
TECHNIQUE   39
OBSERVATIONS   40
CODA   41
EARLY CONSIDERATIONS OF GASTROSCOPY   42
ROSENHEIM OF BERLIN   44

Chapter 3 | From Technology to Vision   46
INTRODUCTION   46
ELECTRICITY   46
THE ROLE OF EDISON   49
LENSES AND OPTICS   50

Chapter 4 | The Metamorphosis-Rigid to Flexible (1900-1930)   55

Introduction   55

Open Tube Instruments   55

Rigid Tubes with Optical Systems   56

Flexible Tubes Straightened After Introduction   57

The Introduction of Flexibility: 1911-1932   58

The Schindler Gastroscope   59

The Semi-Flexible Endoscope   62

Heinrich Lamm   64

Section III | Of Men and Machines   67

Chapter 1 | Rudolf Schindler   68

Early Days   69

Munich 1920   71

Georg Wolf   72

The Lens Problem   74

The Chicago Transfer   75

The New World   76

Twilight Days   78

Epitaph   79

Chapter 2 | American Gastroscopy   80

Cameron and Streifeneder   82

The Final Legacy   84

Chapter 3 | Broadening the Horizon   85

Esophagoscopes of the Semi-Flexible Era   85

Biopsy or Operating Gastroscope   87

Endoscopic Photography   89

Section IV | The Beginning of the Future   93

Chapter 1 | Hirschowitz and Fiber Optics   94

Chapter 2 | Video endoscopy   98

Chapter 3 | Endoscopic Retrograde Cholangio-pancreatography   99

Chapter 4 | Colonoscopy   102

Chromoendoscopy and Magnification Endoscopy   106

Chapter 5 | Laparoscopy   108

Chapter 6 | Percutaneous Endoscopic Gastrostomy   III

Chapter 7 | Endoscopic Ultrasound (EUS)   II2

Section V | *Endoscopic Societies*   II5

THE SCHINDLER - SCHIFF INITIATIVE   II6
THE FOUNDATION OF THE CLUB   II7
THE FIRST MEETING   II8
THE EARLY DAYS   I20
FROM CLUB TO SOCIETY   I23
THE ISSUE OF TRAINING REQUIREMENTS   I24
THE SECOND AND THIRD DECADES (1951-1971)   I25
THE FIBER AND THE FUTURE   I26
THE EXPANSION OF HORIZONS   I26
WORLD ORGANIZATION FOR DIGESTIVE ENDOSCOPY (OMED)   I27
SCHINDLER AND THE SOCIETY   I28
THE CORRIDORS OF POWER: 1971-1981   I29
PUBLIC AWARENESS   I30
HISTORY AND EDUCATION   I3I
ADMINISTRATIVE MECHANISM   I32
FROM BULLETIN TO JOURNAL   I32
1981-1990   I33
1991 - 2000   I34

Section VI | *The Future*   I37

References   I42

FOREWORD

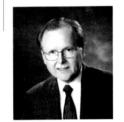

J. T. Frakes

New beginnings foster retrospection. As we start a new century, indeed a new millennium, a mood of reflection is pervasive. Therefore it is appropriate that this book be produced at this time of the millennial epoch. Given the visual nature of endoscopy, it is somewhat surprising that such a graphic pictorial tribute has never before been assembled. This book is timely and true to the subject. Irvin Modlin has created a work which chronicles the history of gastrointestinal endoscopy through text and stunning visual images.

The history of endoscopy has its origin in the 1806 attempt at cystoscopy by Phillip Bozzini using a tin tube, wax candle and mirror. The technical challenges posed then — anatomy, materials, and radiant energy (usually light) to produce a visible image — remain with us. The evolution from rigid endoscopes to semi-flexible instruments to fiberoptic instruments to electronic (video) endoscopy has been accomplished through the collaborations of professional and artisan, physician and engineer, clinician and scientist. Progress has occurred in slow steady increments interrupted by dramatic surges. With this evolution has come an increased ability to diagnose and treat illness — to benefit the patient. From Bozzini, Kussmaul, and Mikulicz, to Schindler and Hirschowitz, to Overholt, Vennes and Waye; from straight tubes to fiberoptics to charged-coupled devices to endoscopic ultrasound, the goal has remained the same: to use technology to better understand patients and to improve their situation, realizing that technology is not an end unto itself but rather a marvelous tool to be used in clinical medicine to advance patient care.

The evolution of digestive endoscopy societies has paralleled that of endoscopic technology. The mission of these societies has been to enhance the quality of patient care by fostering excellence in all aspects of endoscopy. This has been the mission of the American Society for Gastrointestinal Endoscopy (ASGE) as it has promoted the highest standards of endoscopic training and practice, fostered endoscopic research and championed education in gastrointestinal endoscopy. These efforts have nurtured the growth and evolution of both the technology and the ASGE to the point that membership has become synonymous with special skill and expertise. It is appropriate that the ASGE should sponsor this book, along with AstraZeneca and Olympus, its partners from industry. Because it has been an ASGE project, it undeniably gives an American-centric perspective of the history of endoscopy. This view does not diminish the invaluable and oftentimes incomparable contributions of our European and Asian colleagues, which have been noted whenever possible.

Dr. Modlin is to be congratulated for producing this book. It provides perspective, instills pride, and fuels anticipation for our discipline and our technology. As stated by 1985 Rudolf Schindler Award Recipient Dr. William S. Haubrich, "To know the history of endoscopy is to pay tribute to those who have cleared the path we now tread, to understand the impediments that have been overcome, to appreciate more fully the facility we now enjoy, and to point to the prospect of still more marvelous advances to come."

James T. Frakes, M.D., M.S.
Clinical Professor of Medicine
University of Illinois College of Medicine at Rockford
Rockford, Illinois

President
American Society for Gastrointestinal Endoscopy
1999-2000

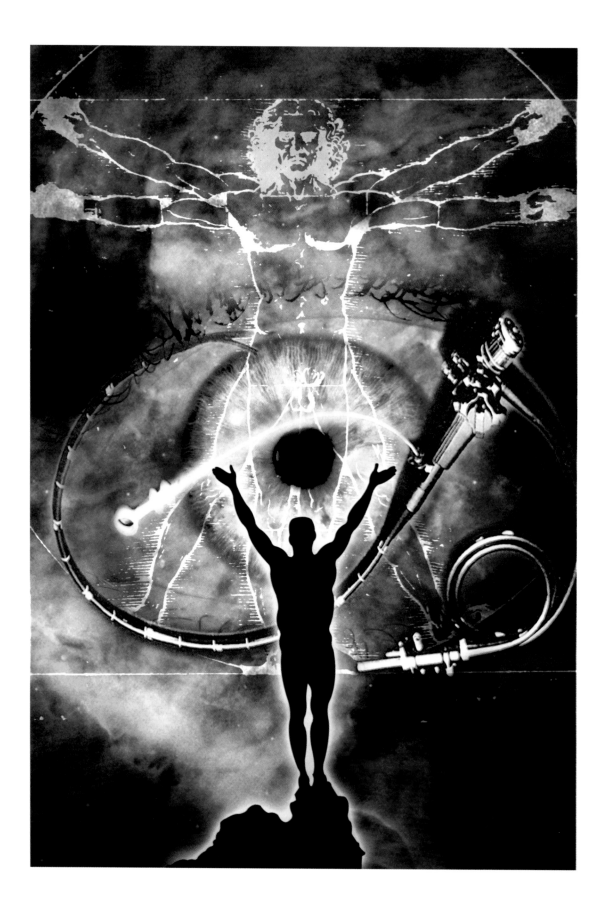

PREFACE

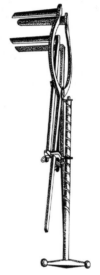

A speculum from the "*House of the Surgeon*" in Pompeii (c. 62-79 AD).

We live in an age when the intellectual expansion of the human mind is constantly incited forward in unremitting vanity to search and explore those qualities, moral and intellectual, proposed to be the fulfillment of life. Under such circumstances the attempt to direct one's gaze backward may be deemed by some to represent a superfluous and even quixotic exercise or endeavor. No doubt the compression of time and the concomitant unreality engendered, as well as the assumptions of ideation and motivation inherent in this exercise distort the warp and woof of the fabric of a man's past and the measure of his achievements. Yet the exploration has merit since to perceive the path past is to dream the path forward and *cognoscenti* as diverse as Einstein and Elliot have opined that "all time past is contained in time present". There is thus no need to fear the chiaroscuro of new thought or be apprehensive of the acceptance of life that in its exploration may threaten a repression of interest in the past. Indeed it seems that this same past characterized by its consummation of lives, societies and systems as well as information and human emotions affords one of the principle foundations from which the present with its plentitude of enthusiasms, knowledge and dreams is arrived at.

Why scrutinize the ideas, motivations and contributions of yesteryear when even those of today are opaque and murky? The validity of such an endeavor memorializes the very existence of those who in the past by virtue of their vision and fortitude provided the impetus whereby the boundaries of knowledge and humanity might be shifted outward. Thus the tale of their lives and achievements serves as a scientific and human benediction of the aspirations both of the intellect and the persona.

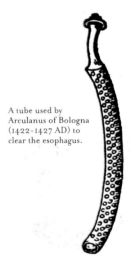

A tube used by Arculanus of Bologna (1422-1427 AD) to clear the esophagus.

> "They shall not grow old,
> As we that are left grow old:
> Age shall not weary,
> Nor the years condemn,
> At the going down of the sun
> And in the morning,
> We shall remember them!"[1]

The recollection of such advances and their associated trials, tribulations and triumphs serves to provide a panorama of distant times against which the brief and fleeting moment of our own present may be gauged. However such perspectives are not easily acquired of those responsible and there is both peril and mystique in an attempt to divine and share even a token understanding of the offerings of the intellect of others. For errors engendered in such assumptions one may only offer the *apologia* inherent in this modest attempt at scholarship.

Given the awe in which man has always held light and vision it is little wonder that endoscopy has attained a place of such primacy in the pantheon of health. Indeed since time immemorial man has feared the darkness and sought to illuminate the deep crevasses of this fear by endlessly seeking to see and understand. Born of a dark and fluid filled chamber, such primitive anxieties were initially allayed by providing fire for the cave and weaponry to repel the marauders of the

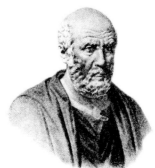

Hippocrates (460-370 BC), the initial descriptor of *dyspepsia*.

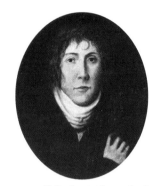

Philip Bozzini (1773-1809) designed the first endoscope (*Lichtleiter*) in Frankfurt in 1805.

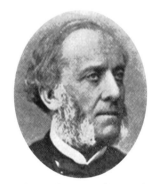

The *Lichtleiter*. The original device courtesy of the archival collection of the American College of Surgeons, Chicago.

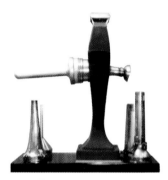

Antonin Desormeux (1815-1881) demonstrated the first functional endoscope (cystoscope) to the *Academie des Sciences* of Paris on November 29, 1853.

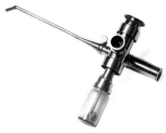

The Desormeux endoscope (courtesy of Musée d'Histoire de la Médicine, L'Ecole d'Medicine, Paris).

flesh. From the opening words of *Genesis* (*and darkness was upon the face of the deep... and the Lord said let there be light...* [2] *{fiat lux}* [3]) to the last moment of life (*and the eyes closed and the light of life departed*) light has endured as a pervasive icon or lodestone of emotional and intellectual importance. Indeed intelligence and curiosity have for long been linked to phrases such as *the light of knowledge* and darkness has been regarded as death, nemesis, disease and an auger of ill. Such subconscious drives may even be implicated in the need to penetrate the outer darkness of space and representative of a deep desire to repel the fear of the *"unseen"*. The exploration of "inner space" can be considered in a similar fashion as an attempt not only to examine the unknown, but also to explore the boundaries of human comprehension and establish the origins of life and the source of death.

Although the earliest sensations of abdominal discomfort were referred to under the Hippocratic generic of *dyspepsia*, their cause was unknown since access to, and knowledge of the interior was prohibited both by lack of medical expertise, religious stricture and fear of divine retribution for meddling with the handiwork of god. Thus in a world illuminated only by fire the cave and home could be lit to repulse carnivores and external perils, but the internal marauders of the flesh (disease) and their locations in the dark recesses of the body were invisible, fearsome and connoted decay and death. Early concepts of the inexplicable nature of illness and its dire consequences (*media vita in morte sumus* [4]) resembled the explanations of external phenomena that could not be visualized. Thus disorders were felt to be the work of deities (inconceivable), divine spirits (invisible) or punishment for sins (dark thoughts or deeds). Relief could best be obtained by prayer (penetrate and illuminate the soul), penance (fasting, flagellation) sacrifice (release of the vital spark) or a by use of a *mithridatum* or diverse array of herbal medications. The cognomen of light was health and the vision of truth and hence cure represented a release from the darkness of sin and mortal decay. Even Descartes, mindful of optical decussation, perceived light and vision to represent the epiphany of the soul and Cartesian doctrine held that perception of the "internal light" of the soul (*Ça mon âme, il faut partir* [5]) to be a necessary human goal.

Frustrated by the inability to perceive the cause of disease, medical curiosity provoked an interest in the examination of the interior via natural orifices. Tubes, specula and digits enhanced by sun, candlelight and mirrors were utilized more than two millennia ago and such incunabula may still be found in the ruins of Babylon and Pompeii. The Romans and Greeks properly regarded the stomach and the sensations emanating from the ingestion of Lucullian repasts and Falernian wine as worthy of their full attention. Thus the murals of Pompeii and the ochre kraters of Atticus attest to the beastly beatitudes afforded the belly and the pleasurable sensations consequent upon a sated stomach and the soaring limbic litany of wine inspired love. The children of the Nile driven by Anubis and a more pyramidal perception of life regarded the lower bowel of more consequence inferring that ill health related to absorption of impurity and that eternal salvation might best be achieved by evacuation. Indeed Irj, a powerful physician of Egypt (2500 BC), was accorded the title of *Shepherd of the Anus*.

Having dispensed with the archaic Phrygian speculation offered by Galenic doctrine, Andreas Vesalius with Flemish candor and acquired Paduan artistry opened the doors of anatomic perception of the viscera. Sadly for the practicing physician, the pristine Calcarine vision could only be acquired *post mortem* and like Bramante's doors the interior of the abdomen remained sealed as Paracelsus pounded upon the parapets of dogma. Such contributions helped disperse the bigotry, dogmatism and mental inertia that characterized the times and the medical illuminati sought to shed light on the interior causes of disease. Cogniscent of Morgagni's *De Sedibus*, P. Bozzini of Frankfurt was the first to peer within the seats of disease and designed an ingenious device (the first endoscope), the *Lichtleiter*, whereby he briefly opened the interior portals of perception. Doomed to an early death by dysentery and Viennese derision, his concept was nevertheless amplified and the *Lux vitae* borne forward. With Gallic flair Pierre Segalas and Antonin Desormeaux of Paris addressed the bladder followed by John Fisher of Boston and Francis Cruise of Dublin as "uranoscopy" progressed to cystoscopy. Disdaining the barber's pursuit of water and stone, Adolf Kussmaul in Freiburg sought the counsel of sword swallowers and became the first to peer beyond the pharynx and Killian's dehiscence. Prescient and ingenious in his use of tubes to divine the mysteries of the humble organ and its reservoir, he saw darkly within the esophagus and stomach before departing this field to pursue the vagaries of respiratory rhythm. The urologist Max Nitze and his engineering colleague Josef Leiter in Vienna, having designed an eminently usable cystoscope, failed to adequately adapt it for gastric usage being apparently unmindful of the navigational differences that distinguished urethral and esophageal anatomy. Disrupted by the fierce enmity of their disagreement in regard to intellectual primacy, Leiter sought to widen the scope of his endeavors and embraced the visionary Slavic surgeon, Johann von Mikulicz-Radecki. Together they sought to explore the northern orifice and seek safe passage to the stomach. Within a decade a functional esophagoscope and gastroscope had been produced and the blind tubes of Fabricius of Aquapendente and Thomas Willis (of cerebro-circular fame) were relegated to history. Buoyed by the electrical contributions of Gustav Trouvé and subsequently Thomas Edison, Leiter produced the pan-electroscope and lo "all became clear." *Fin de siecle* Europe embraced the ideology of Ismar Boas of Berlin, who had laid the foundations of gastroenterology and possessed of lighted, albeit rigid probes, physicians sought diligently to identify the visceral diseases which Theodor Billroth, Bernard Langenbeck and their colleagues thereupon resected with voracious abandon.

The potent intellectual and fiduciary milieu of the Austro Hungarian Empire and Prussia generated major advances in medicine and science that included the inspiration to further the pursuit of endoscopic goals. Thus Elsner, Rosenheim, Sussman, Korbsch and a host of intellectually and technically gifted physicians devised instruments to view the pathology that had previously been only guessed at, while Rudolf Virchow and his colleagues deliberated on the nature of the lesions. Unfortunately lighting, instrument rigidity and optical inadequacy prevailed and despite the prismatic vision of Michael Hoffman and the flexible designs of Georg Wolf for Sussman, vision remained dim and perforation a peril. Aggrieved by the limitations of vision and concerned by the gratuitous and all-pervasive diagnosis of gastritis ,Rudolf Schindler in Munich provided the impetus for the next step. In concert with the Berlin engineer Wolf, an upgraded gastroscope with safety features as well as suction and adequate vision was produced. Within a decade this rigid chrysalis had undergone a further metamorphosis and the resultant semi-flexible gastroscope emerged to revolutionize the world of endoscopy and silence the sycophants of Sauerbruch and their doom-laden prophecies ("*mit tödlichen Ausgang*") of perforation.

Visibility problems of a different sort abrogated further progress in German endoscopy as the advent of the Third Reich obliterated many of the medical *cognoscenti* and Schindler himself

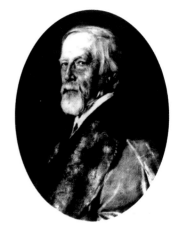

Adolf Kussmaul (1822-1902) pioneered the introduction of gastric aspiration and undertook the first esophagoscopy in 1868.

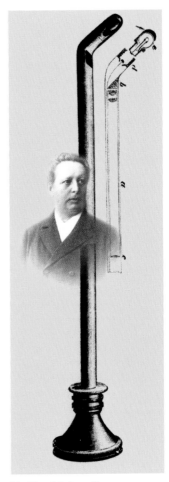

Max Nitze (1848-1906) developed the first effective endoscope with J. Leiter in 1877.

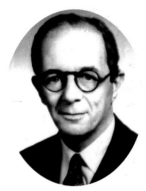

Rudolf Schindler (1888-1968), a
peripatetic polymath and clinician *par
excellance*, who developed the first semi-
flexible gastroscope with G. Wolf in 1932
and in 1941 orchestrated the foundation
of the American Gastroscopic Club.

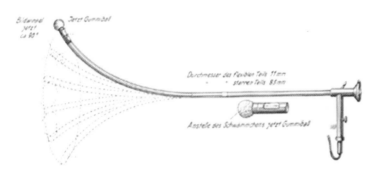

The Schindler-Wolf semi-flexible
gastroscope, c. 1932.

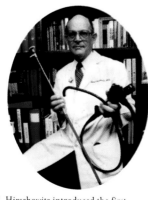

B. Hirschowitz introduced the first
fiber optic endoscope in 1957 in
collaboration with L. Curtiss.

after a six-month sojourn in Dachau immigrated to Chicago. Undaunted by his ignominious
eviction his charisma and ingenuity catalyzed the establishment of the American Gastroscopic
Club in 1941 and thereby engendered a New World renaissance in the utility of gastroscopy.
Propelled by powerful practical and intellectual momentum the society grew rapidly in strength as
its bulletin, scientific meetings and teaching seminars empowered physicians to recognize the diagnostic and therapeutic advantages of appropriately performed endoscopy. Numerous individuals
including Benedict, Janeway, Chevalier Jackson, Howard, Weiss, Katz, Renshaw, Einhorn and
Kirsner provided diverse input that ensured the development of a powerful platform for the evolution of American endoscopy.

In 1957 on a snowy morning in Colorado at the annual meeting of the American
Gastroscopic Society, Basil Hirschowitz demonstrated the utility of fiber optic gastroscopy and
illuminated the dawn of a new era. Although the dream and beauty of bending of light had originated with Daniel Colladon and the fountains of Paris, it was the appreciation of the scientific
concepts initially addressed by Heinrich Lamm, Harold Hopkins and Narinder Kapany that permitted Basil Hirschowitz and Larry Curtiss to finally turn the corner. Indeed Newton's epic
paraphrase of Lucan in Didacus Stella *"Pigmei gigantum
humeris impositi plusquam ipsi gigantes vident"*[6] would never be
more appropriate than in the visual context of endoscopic science. Within a decade the fiberoptic endoscope had entered the pantheon of medical deities
and much as the Greeks worshipped the gods of
Olympus, so did the device and its innumerable
transmutations become venerated amongst gastroenterologists. Indeed as the rising sun illuminates a new
landscape and provides the promise of infinite possibilities, so too did the benders of light perceive a greater future. In a twentieth century version of the intrepid navigators of Prince Henry
rounding Cape Bojador and perceiving a new-world, so did a generation of innovative and daring
endoscopists plot a novel course beyond the pylorus and the sphincter of O'Byrne.

Fiber optic endoscopy amplified and expanded at an exponential rate as both physicians and
corporate technology combined to allow endoscopists and patients to profit from their ability to
see further and do more. The gastroscope was followed by the duodenoscope and it in turn by the
esophagoscope and each augmented by permutations and commutations in flexion and viewing
capacity. McCune arduously visualized the papilla of Vater and Wirsung's duct yielded unwillingly
to the cannula before Oddi's legacy finally capitulated to the currents (high frequency) of
Meinhard Classen and Keichi Kawai. With Carthaginian ingenuity Luciano Provenzale of
Cagliari probed the colon using a pulley propelled gastroscope to attain Tulp's valve, as Bergein
Overholt mastered the rectosigmoid junction and proved that the haustral domain could be safely
broached. Undeterred by Lavoisier's prophets of gaseous implosion and sanguine torrents,
Hiromi Shinya and William Wolff ignored *Atropos* and polypectomized with abandon while Cotton,
Siegel, Salmon Geenen and Oi ballooned, papillotomized, lithotripted and dilated *in excelsior*. In
the far distance the dirge of the demise of open surgical intervention played softly as the lights
slowly dimmed in the operating rooms of the mavens of Mayo.

Dreaming of ever better illuminating the inner darkness and determined to vault beyond the pixel, the caduceus of fiber bundles and lenses yielded to charge coupled devices, computer enhanced imagery and video endoscopy. Motherboards and linear arrays brought the Merlinesque skills of electronic technology to the palaces of the patients and the houses of endoscopy hummed as the circuitry of the "new sight" danced with abandon upon the screens of endoscopic imagination. Almost anything could be seen and there was little that could not be sampled as waves of sound, light and electromagnetic fields bathed the lumen and its vast roseate littoral. Vision beyond surface supplanted the known boundaries of the mucosa as magnification became amplified by dye enhancement and fluorescence spectroscopy superseded chromoendoscopy. Fibrosis and scarring yielded to plastic stents and memory metals, while balloons, tubes, snares and biological liners besieged the waning tide of the acid rain, vanquished the polyp denuded mucosa and rendered the channels of the liver acalculous.

Reader as you next gaze at the glimmering image on the screen and ponder the deep mysteries of the roseate inner life, spare a brief thought for those who placed it there and entrusted to you so wonderful a legacy. Be mindful of their trials, tribulations and travails and seek not to forget that behind the low hum of the circuitry they too were persons (just like you) of ardor, pride and hunger. Let not the pixels of the present blind your vision to the powers of posterity and heed the admonishment that ours is but a brief view of an eternal vision and that all is vanity. One brief biopsy and the screen is dark....

> For in and out, above, about, below,
>
> 'Tis nothing but a magic shadow-show,
>
> Played in a Box whose candle is the Sun,
>
> Round which we Phantom Figures come and go [7]

Irvin M. Modlin

Principe di Savoia, Milan

March, 14th, 2000

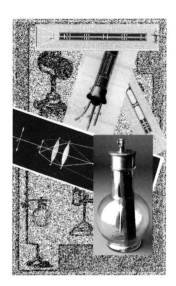

Although clinicians provided the impetus for the development of endoscopy, little would have been achieved without the intense collaboration of mechanical and optical engineers and instrument makers. The resolution of the problems of flexibility, illumination and image transmission initially defied the best minds of two generations.

1. L. Binyon. For the Fallen, st. 4.

2. Pentateuch, First Book of Moses

3. Light of Life, The Vulgate

4. In the midst of life, we are in death.

5. So, my soul, a time for parting, Descartes

6. "Pigmies standing on the shoulders of the giants can see further than the giants themselves". Lucan, Didacus Stella (AD 55).

7. The Rubaiyat of Omar Khayam, 1460 AD. Edward Fitzgerald translation 1941.

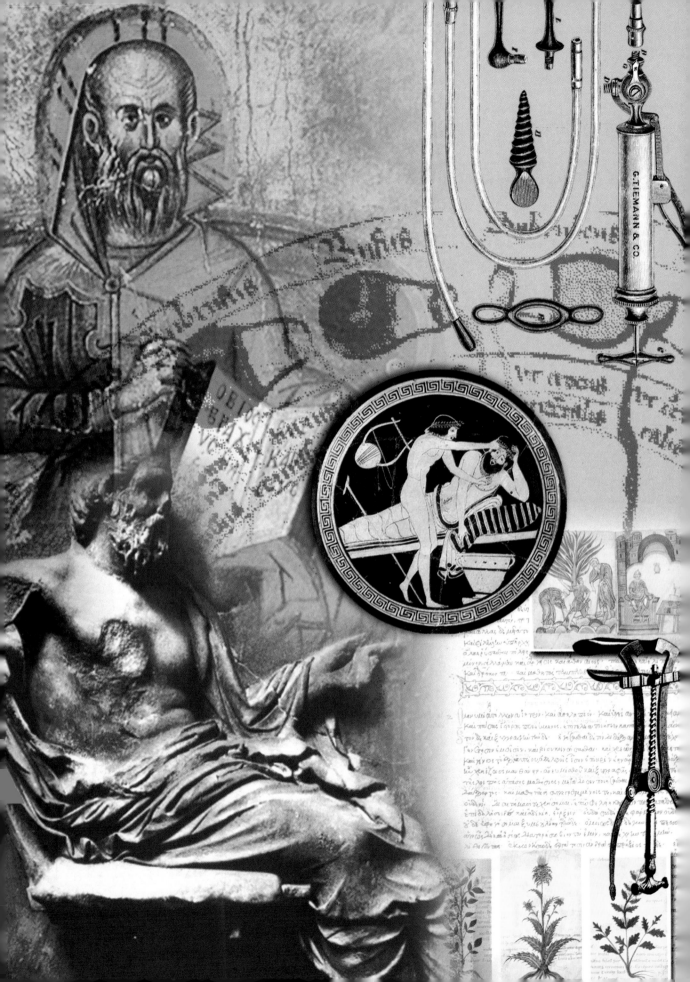

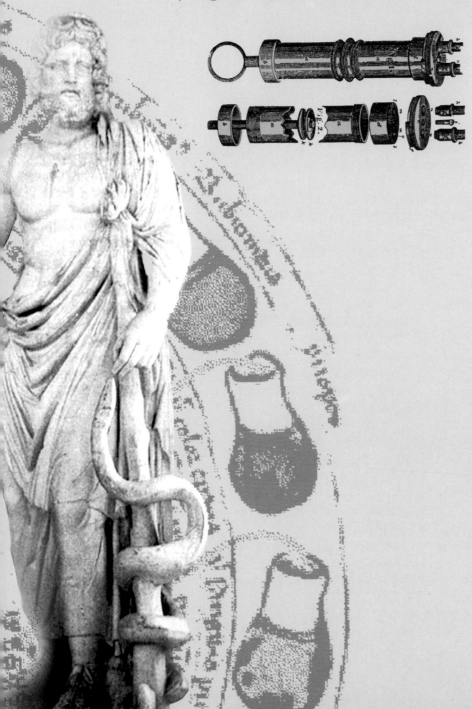

Overview
of the Origins
# of Gastroenterology

CHAPTER I | *A Brief History of Gastroenterology*

In the 17th century the causes of dyspepsia were ill understood and arcane texts still proposed diverse herbal remedies emanating from the work of Dioscorides (c.60 ACE). Von Helmont, an Iatrochemist of Brussels (*top right*) believed that spirits (*archei*) resided in the stomach while Paracelsus in Salzburg (*center*) railed against contemporary dogma, burnt medical books in public and proposed the presence of a *acetosum ensurinum* (hungry acid) in the stomach.

ALTHOUGH THE EARLIEST conceptions of man as related to disease invoked a consideration of divine influences such as the sun, moon and stars, it soon became apparent that some aspects of health were intimately linked to diet. In this respect it was apparent that the ingestion of certain types of food and drink and some bodily activities were closely associated with feelings of profound well being and good health. Thus the ingestion of certain substances not only promoted a sense of bonhomie, but also engendered complex psychic sensations of pleasure and gratification. Whereas absence of water, food and wine as well as lack of sleep and over work generated perceptions of unhappiness and even discomfort. Since the majority of such sentiments related directly to the belly, it was little wonder that the abdomen, and the stomach in particular, became a site to which early man directed substantial attention.

Digestion itself was regarded by Hippocrates (460-370 B.C.E.) as a process akin to cooking or coction and referred to as *pepsis*. Abnormalities of digestion were variously grouped together as dyspepsis, apepsis and even polypepsis and connoted a variety of disease states generously regarded as representative of symptoms due to digestive abnormalities. Given the observation that cooking was related to heat, the clinical symptoms of fever and sweating were thus also held to be related to abnormalities of internal coction. It was therefore widely accepted and self-evident that good food and a sound digestion were absolute necessities to ensure a healthy and productive life.

Abnormalities of digestion or sensations that were unpleasant and located in the abdominal cavity were initially regarded as the results of bad humors or possession by evil spirits or *archei*. Initial concepts of treatment included the avoidance of certain foods, the imbibition of various kinds of waters and extracts of herbs and roots. The development by Pedanius Dioscorides (40-90 A.C.E.) of a rational basis for herbal therapeutics was followed by the introduction of a diverse array of remedies

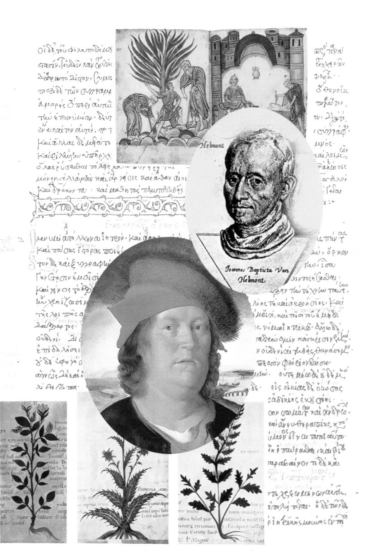

some possessed of known active substances and others simply divine inspirations of bizarre mixtures (*mithradatum*). The fact that the repertoire of symptoms for the gastrointestinal tract was relatively limited (nausea, vomiting, colic, diarrhea, constipation and distention) did not obviate the development of a myriad of extracts, elixirs and homeopathic remedies each guaranteed to alleviate all symptoms and fructify the life of the recipient.

Although the heart, lungs and brain were recognized to be vital, especially in terms of traumatic events and loss of life, it was the abdomen and the stomach in particular which played an ongoing role in the perpetuation of feelings of good health and well-being. Indeed, the sensations of hunger and its abolition were as critical a feature of early behavior as was the primal drive of sexual satiation and procreation.

Thus the stomach became regarded as a critical purveyor of pleasure given its role in the assimilation of food and wine and its obvious association with the post cibal sexual endeavors prompted by the mutual and synergistic pleasures of the table and the reclinium. Indeed through the ages poets, philosophers and gourmands from Catullus to Montaigne and Savarin have noted that few feelings are more powerful than the considerations of pleasure invoked by the oral intake of food and wine, and the consequent sensations of limbic languor. The fact that almost as great a pleasure was derived by the evacuation of the bowels further enhanced the importance of the digestive tract in the consideration of feelings of well being. Thus the exquisite awareness of early man with the pleasures of defecation and the associated sensations of relief resulted in much attention being devoted to such activities. The medical

In a world illuminated only by fire and a hunger for knowledge, the pleasures of food and procreation were of paramount importance. Scenes from an ancient Greek *krater* (*bottom right*) and Roman life (*center*) attest to the commodious nature of the *reclinium* in the pursuit of digestive fulfillment. The sumptuous Venetian banquet of the 18th century (*left*) barely predates the gastronomic raptures of Brillat Savarin, but the finery and pomp devoted to dining exquisitely reflect the continuing recognition of the sensations of well being accorded to gastric and limbic stimulation.

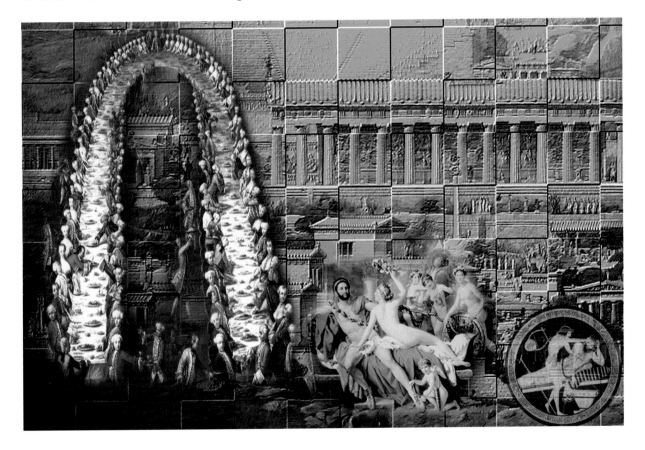

4

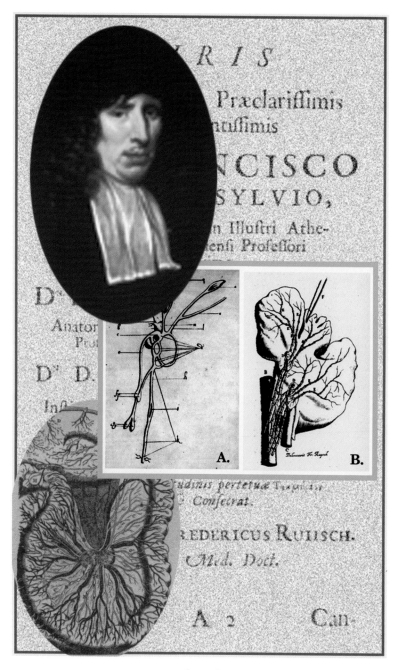

G.Asselli (1581-1626)
and thereafter F. Ruysch
(1638-1723) *(top left)*
delineated the course
of the mesenteric
lymphatics, defined
their valves and
thereby annihilated
the vacuous notion
propounded in 1650
by Louis de Bils
of a circulatory
cardio-mesenteric gyrus
(center left)
implicated in the
process of digestion.

belief that this process was also of importance in ridding the body of noxious agents led to a significant focus on flatus and anal activity. Indeed the tranquillity pursuant upon gaseous discharge and a painless and smooth bowel evacuation was deemed of so much medical significance that considerable therapeutic endeavor was devoted to this area.

The subsequent advent of dissection (A.Vesalius 1514-1564) with the elucidation of precise anatomic structure and relationships both abetted and mutated the world of speculation and conjecture regarding the nature of the function of the abdominal organs and their relation to digestion. Early Iatromathematic concepts (G. Baglivi 1668-1706, G. Borelli 1608-1679, W. Pitcairn 1711-1791) even proposed that the entire digestive system was a mechanical device whereby the teeth were scissors, the stomach a fermenting tank and the intestines transport tubes directed to the septic tank of the cloaca. The counterpart to such proposals was provided by the Iatrochemical doctrine (J. van Helmont 1577-1644, H. Boerhaave 1668-1738) that held that a variety of chemical agents were produced at each site and variously responsible for the processing of food prior to its assimilation.

Although the function of the liver was a source of disputation, T. Bartholin (1616-1680) unceremoniously dismissed the aged Galenic concept of blood formation and proposed a definitive role for the organ in digestion and detoxification. Similarly Regnier de Graaf (1641-1673) proved the pancreas to be a secretory gland, although he erroneously supported F. de la Boe Sylvius (1614-1672) in the notion that it produced a digestive acid. Thus, by the end of the 18th century, a good deal was understood of the basic elements of the digestive process and it was apparent that the secretions of the ductile glands including the salivary, pancreatic and hepatic were critical participants in the processing of food. It might be inferred that while the detailed Paduan anatomical drawings of Vesalius had led to a clear understanding of structure, it was in the Netherlands that the first physiologic concepts of digestive function were satisfactorily addressed. Even A. von Haller (1708-1777) of Bern, whose text on physiology was deemed by Sir William Osler (1849-

1919) to be the gateway to modern thought, was trained at Leiden prior to transferring his intellectual benificence to Göttingen. What remained was the need to firstly correlate function and particularly abnormal function with pathology and secondly to develop a rational therapeutic approach. Clinicians such as Boerhaave of Leiden and subsequently his pupil G. van Swieten (1700-1772) in Vienna promulgated this doctrine widely and ensured that bedside teaching became a regular feature closely interfaced with not only didactic lectures, but also post mortem correlation.

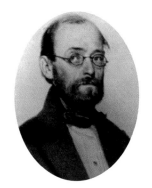

C. Rokitansky, Vienna (1804-1881)

The next major step in the understanding of the gastrointestinal tract involved the establishment of anatomic pathology as a tool, whereby the causation of symptomatology might be directly linked to a disease state. The first definable pathologic information was provided by T. Bonet in his *"Sepulchretum"* of 1679, and thereafter by G. Morgagni (Padua, 1682-1771), J. Cruveilhier (Paris, 1791-1873), C. Rokitansky (Vienna, 1804-1878) and finally by R. Virchow (Berlin, 1821-1902). The meticulously detailed descriptions of innumerable cases (more than 30,000 from Rokitansky alone) produced information that enabled a precise correlation of the symptoms with the autopsy findings.

In this way clinicians became able to predict the underlying pathological process based upon the elucidation of the clinical presentation. So skilled were individuals such as J. Skoda (1805-1881) of the Allgemeine Krankenhaus in Vienna that diagnosis became an obsession and therapeutic nihilism supervened. Cogniscent of the appalling lack of effective treatment, many physicians were satisfied simply with the establishment of a diagnosis and left the outcome of the disease to divine providence. The elaboration of Leeuwenhoek's microscopic design and the further development of lenses provided insight into the more subtle aspects of disease. The microscopic evaluations by Marcello Malpighi (1628-1694) and much later Rudolf Virchow provided for the further delineation of the more detailed aspects of both structure and pathology.

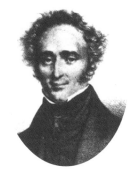

J. Cruveilhier, Paris (1791-1873)

The subsequent contributions of Robert Koch (1843-1910), Louis Pasteur (1822-1895), T. Escherich (1857-1911) and K. Shiga (1870-1957) to the appreciation of a bacterial cause of gastrointestinal disease resulted in the development of knowledge designed to not only identify pathogens but also eradicate such agents. Nevertheless this information was initially of little benefit to patients, since it was either obtained post mortem or adequate antimicrobial therapy was unavailable. Surgery as a therapeutic option was for the most part too quixotic to contemplate (no less an authority than Bernard Naunyn, 1839-1925, considered it to be nothing more than an autopsy in vivo) and targeted specific pharmacotherapy but a dream.

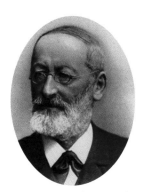

R. Koch, Berlin (1843-1910)

By the second half of the nineteenth century advances in biological chemistry and science led to progression in the discernment of function. In particular the elucidation of the nature of the diverse secretory products of the various parts of the gastrointestinal tract led to the exploration of the regulation of secretion. Ivan Pavlov (1849-1936) initially defined the neural regulation (c. 1900) of secretory and motor function and was followed soon thereafter by the contributions of Sir William Bayliss (1860-1924) and E. Starling (1866-1927), who identified chemical messengers and demonstrated their ability to excite response at a distance (c. 1902).

Such advances were amplified by developments in organ patho-physiology as J. Edkins (1863-1940) described gastrin and J. Langley (1852-1925) pepsin, while A. Einhorn (1856-1917), J. Hemmeter (1864-1931) and F. Krause (1856-1937) vari-

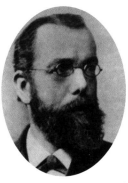

T. Escherich, Vienna (1857-1911)

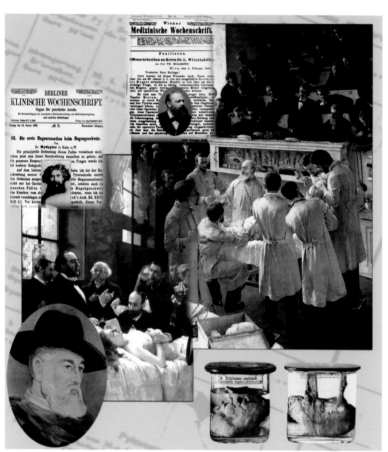

Theodor Billroth in his newly opened operating room in the Allgemeine Krankenhaus, Vienna (A. F. Seligman, 1899). Although the painting was criticized in Vienna, it was acclaimed at the World fairs of Chicago and Madrid (bronze medals) and received gold medals in London and Berlin. The depiction of the operation is accurate and represents a neurectomy for trigeminal neuralgia undertaken on an elderly man. As the primogenitor of gastric surgery, one may whimsically regard Billroth as the first to address the Gut Brain axis. Böttcher hands a scalpel to Billroth while Heidenthaller holds the scissors. The head of the patient is held by Winter and Anton Eiselsberg is the anesthetist, while Beck holds the legs should the patient stir. The painter, A.F. Seligman, is seated at the extreme right of front row. At the far left of the same row sits Karl Theodor, Duke of Bavaria, who frequently attended the lectures of Billroth.

ously explored gastric and duodenal secretion. The advent of W. Roentgen (1845-1923) and his X-rays prompted W. Cannon (1871-1945) to study motility, while bismuth and barium facilitated the skills of G. Bucky (1880-1963), G. Holzknecht (1872-1931) and R. Carman in the diagnosis of gastrointestinal ulcers and tumors.

This constellation of medical and scientific advances expanded the horizons of understanding of gastrointestinal disease to the extent that in 1896 the proposal by Ismar Boas (1858-1938) of Berlin that gastroenterology should be regarded as a separate discipline was well received.

Although rational therapy had advanced somewhat, the early 20th century exhibited few defined forms of pharmacological intervention other than opiates, analgesics, mercury and belladonna. In this milieu of "therapeutic stasis", the development of anesthesia and antisepsis provided considerable impetus for surgeons to enter the abdominal cavity with a degree of safety not formerly available. Whereas surgery of the gut had previously been limited to dramatic interventions undertaken *in extremis* and with a generally dubious outcome, the peritoneal cavity could now be entered with relative impunity. In Vienna and Berlin, T. Billroth (1829-1894), J. von Mikulicz-Radecki (1850-1905), B. von Langenbeck (1810-1887) and C. Langebuch (1846-1901) respectively, pioneered esophageal, gastroduodenal and gallbladder surgery and their clinics trained a new generation of surgeons skilled in the techniques of resection and anastomosis. Baron B. Moynihan (1865-1936) did likewise in England, while in France J. Pean (1830-1898), H. Hartmann (1860-1952) and M. Jaboulay (1860-1913) amplified the work of T. Kocher (1841-1917) of Bern and A. von Eiselsberg (1860-1925) of Vienna. In the United States W. Halsted (1852-1922), C. Fenger (1840-1902), A. Berg (1872-1950), W. Mayo (1861-1939) and A. Ochsner (1896-1981) epitomized the advances of the New World and surgery became a major consideration in the management of gastrointestinal disease. Nevertheless the major issue for the physician treating abdominal disease remained that of access and identification of disease site and type.

Throughout the ages the issues which defined the management of disease process have been particularly exemplified in the gastrointestinal tract. Thus while physical diagnosis and detailed history taking, combined with clinical experience and knowledge of pathology often generated a working diagnosis, the nature and the site of the lesion were for the most part unknown until either operation or autopsy was undertaken. In this respect it might be said that while the outer space of the body had been explored to its best limits, the inner space was a dark and mysterious cavern inhabited by demons and diseases of which little was known. Early attempts to penetrate the darkness had not moved far beyond the pharynx or the anus and rectum. Although the use of specula was well known both by the early Romans and Egyptians, the limitations imposed by inadequate lighting or instrument design rendered visibility more than a hand's breadth or a candle length within the natural orifices of the body impossible.

The introduction of blind tubes and probes of varying designs and construct provided little diagnostic benefit, although they were of some marginal therapeutic utility in displacing obstructing foreign bodies. In the early 19th century the use of gas lamps and candles with reflectors by P. Bozzini (1773-1809), P. Segalas (1792-1875), F. Cruise (1834-1912) and J. Fischer (1797-1850) allowed for some egress into both the upper and lower gastrointestinal tract. In particular the use of such devices to see within the urethra as well as the rectum and vagina provided some measure of diagnostic information as well as the opportunity for therapy such as lithotripsy and cautery. Fortunately by the mid 19th century engineering techniques had improved to the point that longer tubes capable of direct passage into the esophagus and stomach were available, although their rigidity and the lack of appropriate lighting systems rendered their utility both limited and somewhat dangerous.

Credit must be given to P. Bozzini of Frankfurt for first using a lighting device to look within the bladder and to A. Kussmaul (1822-1902) of Freiburg for attempting to visualize the esophagus and the stomach. Subsequent extrapolations of the various urological systems developed by A. Desormeux (1815-1881) and P. Segalas of Paris, enabled M. Nitze (1848-1906) and thereafter J. Mikulicz (1850-1905) of Vienna to progress in the exploration of the bladder, esophagus and stomach respectively. The ensuing productive relationship that developed among engineers, skilled optical instrument makers and physicians facilitated collaborations that led to the emergence of the early science of endoscopy. Despite frustration at the problems posed by rigidity, inadequate lighting and poor lens systems, it was apparent to the physicians of the turn of the 20th century that exploration of the lumen of the gastrointestinal tract was critical for the further understanding of abdominal disease. The contributions of the great optical, scientific and engineering schools of Vienna and Germany facilitated the development of the critical mechanistic contributions that would promote the internal exploration of the gastrointestinal tract.

The accumulation of gastrointestinal knowledge as well as the interest in the gut that had been engendered by the end of the 19th century fueled the concept that this area of medicine might be regarded as an area worthy of special focus. In this respect the Berlin physician Carl Ewald (1845-1915), and particularly his pupil Ismar Boas, were powerful leaders that influenced physicians in the

Examples of ancient Roman surgical implements (wound probes and lancets) as well as a speculum from the ruins of Pompeii. Most medical thought was originally of Greek and Alexandrian origin, since the Romans thought little of physicians. Ideologues such as Pliny and Cicero considered medical art too be little more than *"Greek puffery"* practiced by foreigners and rogues more skilled in the art of poisons than cures. The assimilation of Greece by the Roman Empire led to the slow acceptance of Grecian medical ideology. The speculum (*top left*) recovered from the House of the Surgeon in Pompeii (c. A.C.E. 62-79) attests to the early fascination and skill in seeking to visualize the interior of the body. Its design would remain almost unchanged until the early 20th century.

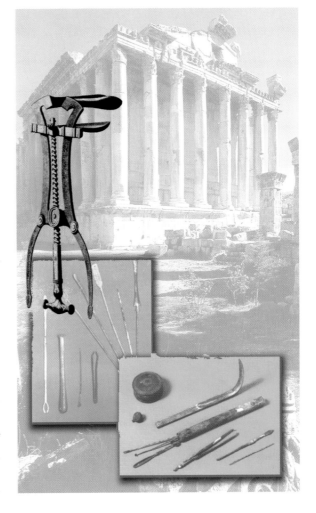

8

establishment of gastroenterology as a separate discipline. Indeed to Boas must be given the credit for founding gastroenterology and establishing the first journal devoted specifically to the topic. His establishment of a clinic specifically for the management of gastrointestinal problems was followed by the publication of a number of textbooks on the subject of the stomach that would attain almost biblical status. Boas emphasized the need for internal exploration of the lumen of the gut and even in the light of the limited early instruments available predicted the future utility of endoscopy.

Prior to Boas' publication of the first textbook solely devoted to the new discipline of gastroenterology (in its entirety), *"Diagnostik und Therapie der Magenkrankheiten"*, printed in Liepzig in two parts between 1890 and 1893, only a few specialized discourses on organs or their disease had been printed. Thus, John of Arderne (1307-1370) had published a treatise on the cure for anal fistula as early as 1376, while G. Stahl (1660-1734) produced a classic work on hemorrhoids in 1730. The 19th century saw the first American discourse on colo-rectal surgery, published by G. Bushe (1793-1836) posthumously in 1837, books on operations for esophageal tumors (A. Middeldorpf 1857) and a work documenting the findings from 7,000 peptic ulcer disease post-mortems (W. Brinton, 1857). Boas' text inspired an explosion of literature and within a decade a number of classic gastroenterological texts, including those by C. Ewald and the American, J. Hemmeter, had been published. Focus on the subject as a whole, rather than specialized areas, had become the norm rather than the exception.

In 1896 W. C. Roentgen in Wurzberg described the X-rays that would provide internal vision of not only body cavities but also, with the advent of bismuth and barium, the very interstices of the gut lumen itself. Similarly the early contributions of Mikulicz, J. Leiter (1830-1892) and Nitze in Vienna in the development of rigid endoscopes were amplified and extended by T. Rosenheim (1860-1910), W. Sternberg, G. Wolf (1873-1938) and finally Rudolf Schindler (1888-1968), who not only introduced novel lens systems, but for the most part overcame the problems of flexibility and illumination. The subsequent application of H. Hopkins (1918-1994) and N. Kapany's work on optics and the development by Basil Hirchowitz and Larry Curtiss of flexible fiber optic endoscope enabled the design of instruments that

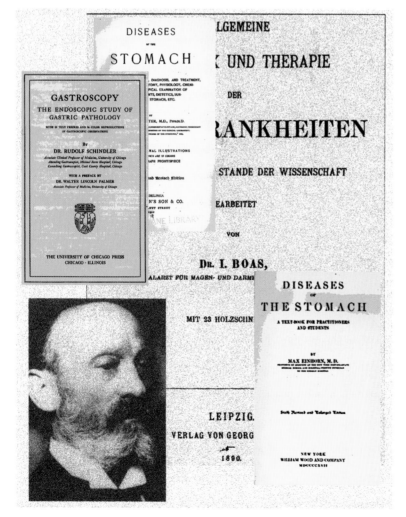

would allow the illumination and vision of the farthest reaches of the bowel. Thus in almost a century the physician had moved from the orifice of a hard steel tube illuminated by candle or gas light to a charge coupled device and video endoscopic monitoring.

This book seeks to recount the tale of how man, having long gazed at the darkness of outer space, has sought to illuminate the darkness of his inner space. The story will wend its way from the earliest blind luminal probing of the ancients through the development of lamps and lenses to a world of fiber optics and lasers. It will document the people and the places as well as the trials and tribulations that have marked the road as light passed from the macula to the mucosa.

1988		Videoendoscopy
1983	Warren/Marshall -	*H. Pylori*
1981	Sachs/Fellenius ---	Proton Pump inhibitors
1973	Black ------	H2 Receptor antagonists
1957	Hirschowitz -----	Fiberoptic endoscope
1932	Schindler/Wolf---	Semi flexible Gastroscope
1922	Schindler -----	Rigid Gastroscope
1910	Dale -----	Histamine
1905	Edkins ------	Gastrin
1902	Elsner -----	Rigid Gastroscope
1902	Bayliss/Starling --	Chemical messengers
1902	Kelling -----	Laparoscopy
1900	Pavlov ------	Nervism
1896	Boas -------	1st Digestive Disease Clinic
1895	Roentgen -----	X Rays
1881	Mickulicz ----	Esophagoscopy/Gastroscopy
1881	Billroth -------	Gastrectomy
1879	Nitze/Leiter ----	Cystoscope
1870	Lister -------	Antisepsis
1868	Kussmaul -----	Gastroscopy
1853	Desormeaux ----	Cystoscope
1829	Beaumont -------	Gastric Digestion
1827	Segalas -------	Urethrocystoscope
1823	Prout -------	Gastric Acid=HCL
1805	Bozzini --------	Lichtleiter
17__	Boerhaave -------	Ruptured Esophagus
16__	De Graaf --------	Pancreatic Fistula
1660	Borelli -------	Iatromathematics
1620	van Helmont -----	Iatrochemistry
1560	Vesalius --------	Anatomy
1200	School of Salerno --	Surgery
200 AD	Galen --------------	Hepatic Hegemony
400 BC	Hippocrates -----	*Pepsis*

A brief time line of some of the notable events and individuals involved in the history of gastroenterology, with especial reference to the development of the discipline of endoscopy.

CHAPTER 2 | *The Development of the Stomach Tube*

THE CONCEPT OF access to the interior of the gut had long fascinated both patients and their physicians. At first the requirements were simple and based upon the need to either remove *per os* foreign objects that had become lodged or to open up the lower passages when feelings of distention and obstruction were perceived to be present. Thus early attempts at medication were targeted at either promotion of emesis or acceleration of defecation and purges and clysters were the order of the day.

With time however the frustration and impatience of physicians with such unpredictable intervention led to efforts to gain more direct access to the interior of the gut. The ingenious development of a diverse variety of tubes was first aimed at therapy either for removing blockages, dilating strictures or providing sustenance. After recognizing the limitations of the finger or the feather, the concept of using tubes to enter the alimentary tract represented the initial early and important impetus in promoting access to the interior. At first these were rigid and introduced blindly, but the discovery of more pliable agents, functional light sources and thereafter lenses led to increased flexibility and better visibility. Thus therapeutic applications initially preceded diagnostic usage and only after the advent of fiber optic technology was parity regained. To fully understand the evolution of the science of endoscopy it is useful to examine the strides along the path that have been undertaken as man has moved from blind bougies to flexible fiber optics.

EMPTYING THE STOMACH

It had long been recognized that a full stomach generated a feeling of discomfort and in many cases inhibited eating and interfered with exercise. This was partic-

A modification of the *Rose Garden of Heliogabalus* by Sir Alma Tadema. Gargantuan meals of the Lucullian school of Roman cuisine culminated in massive gastric distention and precluded further ingestion as well as limiting the aptitude for post cibal debauchery. A discerning host would therefore provide peacock feathers for posterior pharyngeal stimulation and the initiation of emesis, thereby allowing a guest to proceed with the further activities of the evening. The exquisite meals of lark tongues, Caspian caviar, ostrich brain and Falernian wine provided by the Roman Emperor Heliogabalus culminated in a variety of digestive sensations. These ranged from ethanol induced languor to an ecstatic gastric epiphany or even demise. Should there be any perception on the part of the Emperor that the guests were unhappy, hidden ropes supporting the roof of the tent were pulled and the diners suffocated beneath many tons of rose petals. Those who survived might avail themselves of the peacock feathers provided to stimulate self-emesis and thereafter resume further gluttony.

ularly disadvantageous in early history when large complex banquets were the custom and post prandial exotic activities an important part of social intercourse. A perusal of the cooking texts of Apicius or the dinner descriptions of Trimalchio provide clear evidence that a Roman banquet was often little more than a gastric stress test. Since decorum dictated that the entire banquet be completed, skill at the art of self-emesis was necessary both to prevent the after effects of an overloaded stomach as well as to ensure meritorious participation in the remainder of the evening's activities. While emetics were initially employed to generate gastric emptying, nausea and incomplete voiding accompanied low dosages, while excessive usage culminated in ongoing emesis despite the stomach having already been emptied. A simple introduction of the finger into the back of the throat was deemed immodest and from the time of the Emperor Claudius, dinner guests were either provided with a "pinna" or a vomiting feather at the completion of each banquet course.

A further utility of such self-induced emesis was in the rapid evacuation of covertly administered poisons. The application of such ingenuity to obviate the effects of covertly administered poison was circumvented by Agrippina, who poisoned the Emperor Claudius by applying the agent to the feather itself! In the 4th century A.C.E, the master physician Oribasius described a number of methods utilized to produce emesis. These included swinging an individual in a suspended bed; goose feathers dipped in iris or cypress oil, and a variety of herbal combinations. More direct intervention included a digital vomitorium that consisted of a long feather glove, 10 to 12 inches in length, of which the lower two thirds were filled with wood fiber while the upper third remained empty to receive the directing finger of the physician. Presumably this novel device might be regarded as the earliest form of gastric sound.

Although the utility of such instruments decreased as Roman gluttony abated, they were still of some use to physicians who were employed to protect royal personages from would-be poisoners. By the 16th century, Hieronymus Mercurialis had described a more elegant device for the induction of vomiting. This *lorum vomitorium* had initially been described for the treatment of opium poisoning by Scribonius Largus in the 1st century and consisted of a leather strap treated with a nauseating tannic acid-containing substance. The combination of the strap and the chemical when introduced into the esophagus resulted in emesis.

INSTRUMENTATION OF THE STOMACH

The earliest usage for such devices involved the removal of foreign bodies from the esophagus by forcing them into the stomach itself. The first prototypes consisted of short perforated metallic tubes designed to clasp foreign bodies such as fish bones and extract them. In 1493, Johannes Arculanus, professor at Bologna and Padua, described a lead tube for this purpose, but by the 17th century, J. Scultetus (1595-1645) and Giulielmus Fabricius Hildanus (1560-1624) had written extensive manuscripts describing modifications. These ranged from simply constructing the tube of silver to more creative designs that included the attachment of small sponges to the lower end. The device utilized by Hildanus consisted of "a hollow silver bent tube the size of a swan's feather about a foot and a half in length. This tube, which is perforated throughout its length and has a sponge the size of a hazelnut securely attached at its end, is introduced in the esophagus and is utilized with much success in extracting fish bones, small bones, and other foreign objects."

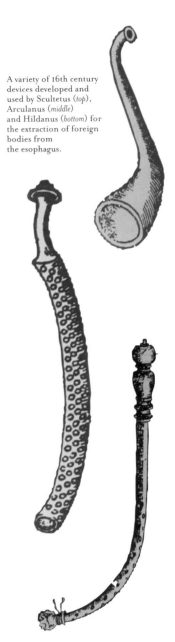

A variety of 16th century devices developed and used by Scultetus (*top*), Arculanus (*middle*) and Hildanus (*bottom*) for the extraction of foreign bodies from the esophagus.

II

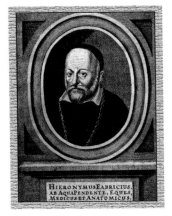

Hieronymus Fabricius
ab Aquapendente (1537-1619)

No less an authority than the great anatomist Hieronymus Fabricius ab Aquapendente (1537-1619) advocated that foreign bodies which could not be extracted using devices of this kind be pushed into the stomach. He further amplified his contributions in this area by not only devising an instrument for this purpose, but also producing a tube that could be utilized for artificial feeding in patients who could not swallow. The device consisted of a silver tube covered with the intestine of a sheep to facilitate its introduction through the esophagus into the stomach. Thus by the 17th century the stomach tube had graduated from its initial use in the removal of foreign bodies or their pulsion into the stomach, to the earliest form of enteral nutrition.

THE STOMACH BRUSH

Ancient wisdom proposed that noxious agents in the stomach provided a general feeling of ill health and were responsible for a diverse array of symptomatology which might range from modest halitosis through lassitude, distension, vomiting, and even fatal decline. The concept arose, therefore, of either purging the stomach by emesis induced by herbal mixtures or alternatively cleansing the stomach. Such cleansing could be undertaken either by the administration of herbal mixtures such as aloes, saffron and myrrh or the use of mechanical devices. By the middle of the

An advert and depiction of the stomach brush as utilized by J. C. Socrates, 1719. The instrument was constructed of strong carefully bound and padded steel wires that were encircled with silk thread. It was 26 inches in length and tipped with a brush of 3 inches in length and 2 in breadth, which was held firm by means of goat or horse hair. To facilitate its introduction, the instrument was slightly bent and carefully soaked in water before swallowing. Socrates suggested that substantial quantities of diluted brandy be imbibed prior to the introduction of the *Magenraumer*!

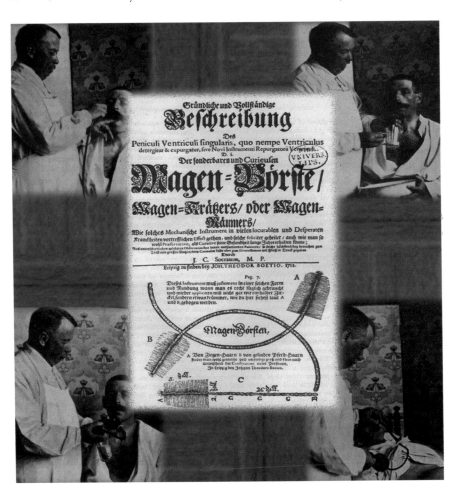

12

17th century a stomach cleanser or brush (*Magenkratzer* or *Magenraumer*) had been devised for direct application to the interior of the stomach.

The stomach brush consisted of a long smooth flexible arched whale bone, two to three feet in length, tipped with an ivory button to which a tuft of silk cord, horse hair or linen was firmly attached. Having been passed through the mouth and esophagus into the stomach, the appropriate cleaning maneuvers were undertaken. As a consequence of these drastic activities, copious vomiting was usually induced and visible evidence of gastric emptying and cleansing was evident to all. So effective was this device that it became known as the "cure" and the instrument was often hidden in monasteries or convents where its usage was regarded as a sacred secret or "*arcanum*".

Such instruments proved so effective in the hands of certain physicians, that they were proposed for usage in even healthy individuals as a prophylactic measure by which means a long life could be attained and all stomach troubles avoided. Indeed the concept acquired such vogue that men of considerable medical stature including L. Heister (1683-1758) supported outrageous statements made by the likes of Socrates who claimed "it appears as if death had laid aside its scythe and instead has had the stomach cleanser placed in its hands".

Although the technique of gastric brushing caused some problems, a number of reports detailed quite clearly its effectiveness in the cure of chronic gastric ailments. Thus in 1649, Rumsey, an English physician, wrote glowing of its effectiveness, as did Sobierus of Paris in 1694. In the same decade the King of Denmark was so taken with the procedure that he personally witnessed a live demonstration of its utility. Most impressive of all, however, is a detailed account of the complete cure of a Russian aristocrat repetitively treated in a convent for "over fatigue and the excessive abuse of alcohol". After large doses of brandy and water, the "*Magenkratzer*" was applied until the stomach was entirely cleansed of mucus, bile, and a clotted foul smelling purulent material had been discharged by mouth. Introduction of the brush was continued on a daily basis for eight days with intermittent nutrition of eggs, soup, and softened chicken. A complete success was pronounced at the end of two weeks and the noble declaring himself cured became so impressed with the treatment that he self administered it for a further 14 years. It is likely that such circumstances actually reflect individuals with various gastric emptying disorders and that the brush either removed a bezoar or alternatively prevented its formation.

Lest it be thought that only the Europeans were involved in such matters, Dapper traveling with the Dutch West Indies fleet in 1673 described a novel treatment he had witnessed amongst the South American Indians. "The Tapagus, a Brazilian tribe, have a remarkable method of cleansing the stomach. They pass a rope made of padded sharp leaves down the throat and into the stomach and then turn and twist it until vomiting and a bloody discharge occurs. The rope is then withdrawn and the stomach is cleansed."

Unfortunately poor results followed prolonged usage of gastric cleansing treatment and a variety of ailments such as esophageal perforation, gastric bleeding and even the development of carcinoma in the stomach led to the technique falling into disuse. Nevertheless the instrument underwent a renaissance and became modified as an upgraded "sound" for the treatment of esophageal disease. Reconstructed in the form of a whale bone sound tipped with a large sponge it thereafter became utilized to treat esophageal obstruction.

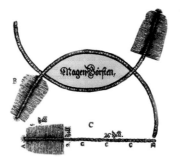

A *Magenkratzer or Magenraumer* (c.mid 17th -18th century). Desperate to alleviate the ill understood symptoms of dyspepsia, even notable physicians such as L. Heister supported rigorous brushing of the stomach with a view to attaining a state of gastric cleanliness.

Lorenz Heister (1683-1758). Probably better remembered for being the first to identify appendicitis (*post mortem*) and introduce the term tracheotomy than for his contributions to gastric hygiene.

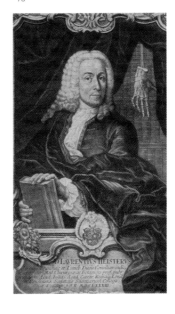

An Esophageal Application

The use of sounds for the dilation of the esophagus became a far more impressive therapeutic application than that generated by the stomach-cleansing vogue. Thomas Willis (1621-1675) reported a patient whose inability to swallow food was so dire that his emaciation had reached a point where even desperate means were worthy of consideration. Willis utilized an esophageal sound covered with a large sponge and not only accomplished a successful dilation of the esophagus but continued the treatment safely for a further 16 years with the patient remaining in good health.

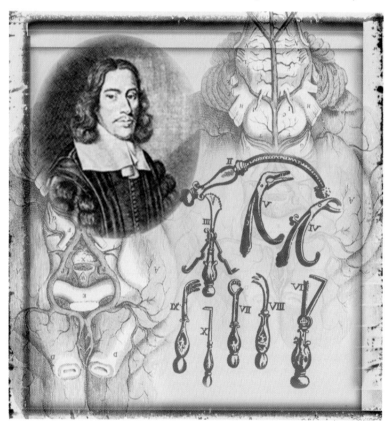

Given the survival time of the patient and the lack of any history of imbibition of a corrosive substance, it is possible that this represents the first successful description of dilation of a benign stricture induced by gastro-esophageal reflux disease. So effective was this form of therapy and swallowing in the management of swallowing problems, that M. Geuns (1735-1817) of Holland in 1784 manufactured a series of sponged tipped ivory olive bougies that were utilized for the treatment of esophageal stenosis. In a book entitled *"Die Krankheiten des Magens"*, Abercrombie reported his use of a silver esophageal sound with an oval knob at its tip for the dilation of esophageal strictures.

Artificial Feeding

It was apparent that if the esophagus was closed the use of an esophageal sound to dilate the stricture was effective. However, in circumstances where the patient could not swallow a different process was required. Thus Hieronymus, Capivacceus and Fabricius ab Aquapendente attempted to devise solutions to this problem. Capivacceus utilized a tube that was introduced through the mouth into the stomach. The upper end was attached to an animal bladder into which the nutritive fluid was inserted prior to expression into the stomach.

Fabricius modified the device by utilizing a small silver tube covered with lamb's intestine that was then inserted through the nose into the esophagus for the purpose of artificial feeding.

These devices developed respectively in Venice and Padua were improved upon by van Helmont and Boerhaave of the Lowlands, who produced flexible catheters of leather that were both easier to introduce and of a greater length. Boerhaave in fact proposed that such tubes might also be utilized not only for introducing nutritive substance, but also antidotes in the event of an individual who had been poisoned and might be unable to swallow.

Thomas Willis (1621-1675) (*top left*) achieved immortality for his description of the arterial circle at the base of the brain. His friend Sir Christopher Wren, who initially practiced as a physician before becoming an architect of hospitals and St Paul's cathedral, undertook the actual drawings of the eponymous circle. Willis was experienced in the use of esophageal sounds to either remove foreign bodies or dilate strictures. His classic description of 16 years of successful esophageal dilation may well represent the first description of achalasia. At the bottom right of the collage are a variety of 17th century devices utilized for the extraction of foreign bodies from the pharynx and esophagus.

Hunter was clearly fascinated with the concept of artificial feeding and in 1793, he further documented a similar application in a manuscript entitled "*A Case of Paralysis of the Muscles of Deglutition cured by an Artificial Mode of Conveying Food and Medications into the Stomach*". The manuscript documents a 50-year-old man who had developed unremitting depression, anxiety and hypochondriasis. "Such was his distress that he awakened each morning with a sense of choking and soon felt a numbness in the whole of his right side, together with a paralysis of the muscles of deglutition which deprived him of the power of swallowing." Hunter devised a hollow flexible tube, which the patient then passed into his stomach twice daily with the purpose of introducing flower of mustard and tincture of valerian. Hunter described the instrument in detail: "a fresh eel skin of rather a small size, drawn over a probang and tied up at the end, where it covered the sponge, and tied again close to the sponge, where it fastened to the whale bone, and a small longitudinal slit was made into it just above this upper ligature. To the other end of the eel skin was fixed a bladder and wooden pipe, similar to what is used in giving a clyster, only the pipe was large enough to let the end of the probang pass into the bladder without freeing up the passage. The probang thus covered was introduced into the stomach and the food and medicines put into the bladder and squeezed down through the eel skin".

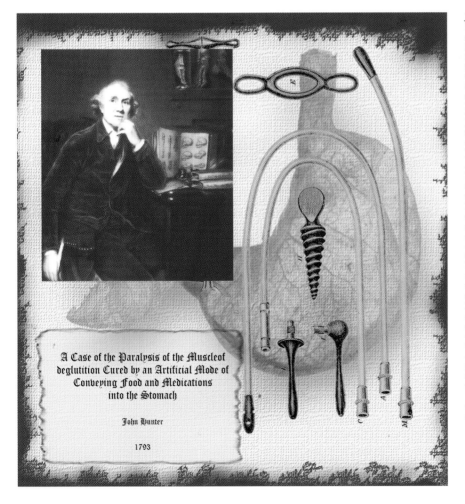

A Case of the Paralysis of the Muscle of deglutition Cured by an Artificial Mode of Conveying Food and Medications into the Stomach

John Hunter

1793

John Hunter of London (1728-1793) was the first surgeon scientist and intellectually explored the structure and function of the body in almost every species available leaving in excess of 50,000 specimens at his death. His friend Sir Joshua Reynolds painted the portrait (*top left*) (Courtesy of the Huntarian Museum of the Royal College of Surgeons of London). In the background is an injected specimen of the stomach from the Huntarian collection and the foreground instruments are of the type utilized to "*sound*" the esophagus.

On March 21, 1776 Hunter delivered a paper entitled "*Proposals for the Recovery of Persons apparently Drowned*". In this essay Hunter amplified Boerhaave's suggestions by describing the use of syringe attached to the hollow bougie or flexible catheter of sufficient length such that it might be introduced into the stomach and "convey stimulating matter into it without affecting the lungs".

TREATMENT OF POISONING

In 1797 Alexander Tertius Monro (1773-1859) provided in his inaugural medical thesis ("*Disputatio Medica Inauguralis de Dysphagia*") a description of the use of a tube and syringe in cases of poisoning.

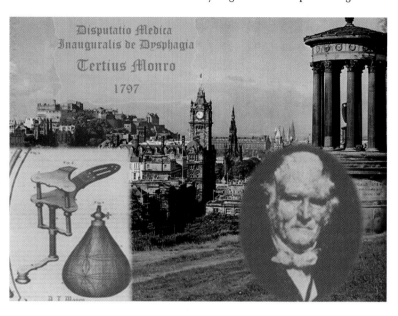

Alexander Tertius Monro (1773-1859) (*bottom right*) was the third successive member of the Monro family to hold the Chair of anatomy in Edinburgh. His thesis *"Disputatio Medica Inauguralis de Dysphagia"* elegantly described the design and use of a tube, syringe, siphon and expandable mouthpiece/tongue depressor (*bottom left*) that had been designed to empty the stomach of ingested poison. This device represented an extrapolation of a similar piece of apparatus first utilized by his father to decompress Highland cattle (Black Angus) suffering from acute gastric distention.

He proposed that the tube could be utilized not only for the extraction of poison from the stomach but also for the introduction of food into the stomach of individuals with severe dysphagia and an inability to swallow. His observations were based on the work of his father, who as early as 1767 had employed a flexible tube in the treatment of cattle, to remove fermenting fluids and gasses from their stomach in instances of great distention. Throughout Europe the utility of stomach tubes was apparent to a number of creative physicians. Thus, apart from the contributions of Hunter of England and Monro of Edinburgh, Baron G. Dupuytren (1777-1835) and C. Renault of Paris had in 1803 not only suggested the use of a flexible tube of sufficient length to reach the stomach, but connected it to a syringe to aspirate swallowed poison. In his great work on toxicology in 1815, M. Orfila (1787-1853) of Paris had cited such Gallic proposals with considerable enthusiasm.

A further French contribution was that of Baron D. Larrey (1766-1842), the Surgeon General of Napoleon Bonaparte. Larrey described in detail the management of a soldier whom he cured of a catastrophic throat wound at the Battle of Aboukir in 1801. Noting the patient to be dying of dehydration in the desert heat since he was incapable of swallowing, Larrey devised a flexible tube that could be passed into the esophagus and allowed the patient to be fed, thus saving his life.

Philip S. Physick (1768-1837), Professor of Surgery at the University of Pennsylvania, provided the American contribution to the use of the stomach tube in the treatment of poisoning. In 1812, he published a paper entitled *"Account of the New Mode of Extracting Poisonous Substances from the Stomach"*. Utilizing a large flexible catheter, he had washed out the stomachs of two three-month-old twins who had been accidentally given an overdose of laudanum by their mother. The technique he utilized entailed injecting a dram of diluted ipecac into the stomach with a syringe and then withdrawing the fluid contents of the stomach repeatedly with instilled warm water. Unfortunately only one of the children was saved and Physick noted that an important issue was the length of time that had elapsed before the removal of the poison. In a subsequent communication the following year, Physick generously acknowledged that Alexander Monro, Jr. of Edinburgh, had in fact previously published his novel proposal. "I, therefore, am happy in having called the attention of the profession to a mode of treatment not before used in this country, at least within my knowledge; but I have now an act of justice to perform, in

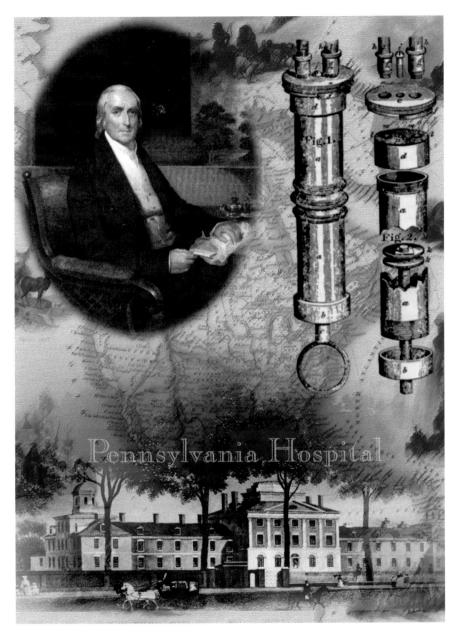

Pennsylvania Hospital

Although the eminent medical historian Fielding Garrison was of the opinion that Philip S Physick (1768-1837) (top left) "wrote nothing of consequence", posterity has nevertheless accorded to him the honorific of "Father of American Surgery". An Edinburgh graduate of 1792 and a pupil of John Hunter, he subsequently became Professor of Surgery at the Pennsylvania Hospital in Philadelphia. In 1812 he published *"An Account of the New Mode of Extracting Poisonous Substances from the Stomach"* and in so doing claimed to have described a novel method of treatment. A year later he was forced to recant this claim when it became apparent that Monro of Edinburgh was the rightful author. Nevertheless he was the first American to use a syringe and tube to wash out the stomach in a case of poisoning. Since the case described was that of twins accidentally overdosed with laudanum by their mother and one died, his mortality was 50%. The syringes and pumps (*top right*) used for the purpose of extracting gastric contents underwent a series of modifications and a series of London physicians including Bush (1822), Jukes (1822) and Mathews (1826), each laid claim to priority of the invention.

describing the merit of the invention to Dr. Alexander Monro, Jr. of Edinburgh who published it in his inaugural thesis in AD 1797. Of this cir-cumstance I was entirely ignorant when I sent you my paper." Since Physick had published his own manuscript in 1812 and had studied in London with John Hunter, his gracious afterthought may have been somewhat disingenuous.

Further argument arose regarding the priority of the discovery of the stomach tube. Thus in 1826, Mathews in a publication entitled *"Description of an Improved Instrument for Extracting Poison from the Stomach with some Statements tending to establish the Validity of Dr. Physick's title to the credit of having invented the Stomach Tube"* further addressed the issue. Mathews described a syringe of his own and provided certificates from three other physicians supporting his primacy. Physick claimed that he recommend-ed the introduction of the tube into the stomach as early as 1802 and that he had initially demonstrated the tube covered with elastic gum in 1805, which had been brought to him by his nephew, Dr. John Dorsey, from Paris. Mathews also criticized E. Jukes and F. Bush of London as well as D. Evans and W. Reed, each of whom had claimed priority for the discovery at this time. In May 1822, Jukes, an English surgeon, had published a paper entitled "*New Means of Extracting Opium from the Stomach*", in which he described an instrument that he called a "stomach pump" for "removing by mechanical agency, poison from the stomach". The apparatus consisted of a flexible tube a quarter of an inch in diameter, two and a half feet in length, tipped with an ivory globe containing several perforations. The other extremity was attached to an elastic bottle filled with warm water and following the introduction of the tube into the stomach the fluid was forced in and out. Such was Jukes' skill that he had successfully experimented on dogs into whose stomach he had introduced laudanum and thereafter irrigated it until the water extracted became clear. To further confirm the efficacy of his treatment, he swallowed ten drams of laudanum and allowed his colleague, Mr. James Scott, to undertake a successful lavage. This performance was repeated in public at Guy's Hospital to the considerable admiration of Sir Astley Cooper (1768-1841).

Although Jukes published his observations in the London Medical and Physical Journal of November 1822, Bush had described a similar technique in September of the same year in the same journal. The latter utilized a flexible tube to enter the stomach but instead of an elastic bottle employed a syringe. Bush termed his apparatus a "gastric exhauster" and as a result a debate of considerable acrimony regard-

Sir Astley Cooper (*top right*) was the doyen of British surgery during the early 19th century and apart from his sartorial elegance recognized as an individual of quixotic intellectual genius. Guy's Hospital (*bottom right*) where he practiced has long been the recipient of widespread acclaim as the origin of numerous medical and scientific advances. Wittgenstein, Bright, Addison, Hodgkin, Gull and a host of intellectual *illuminati* have graced its portals. In 1822, Scott and subsequently Reed demonstrated the use of a Gastric Exhauster (*top left*) to Cooper and convinced him of its efficacy. As a footnote it is worth commentary that William Prout also worked at Guy's and his first description of the presence of hydrochloric acid in human gastric juice (1823) presumably reflects his access to the material provided by these demonstrations.

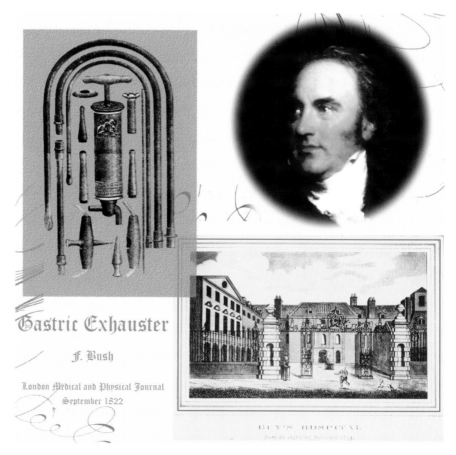

Gastric Exhauster

F. Bush

London Medical and Physical Journal
September 1822

GUY'S HOSPITAL.

ing primacy ensued. Unfortunately for both parties, Evans had in 1817 employed a similar mechanical device with a stomach tube to effect the removal of opium; however, his work was not published until 1823.

Later that year on November 21st, Reed, once again at Guy's Hospital, demonstrated to Astley Cooper and his students a similar but more advanced apparatus for the emptying of the stomach. Mr. Reed had developed a syringe with two valves thus obviating the need for repetitive removal of the syringe during the process of gastric lavage. In 1825, J. Weiss of Germany developed and patented a new pump which he claimed could be used for the emptying of the stomach of poisons, water from drowned persons, or for the presentation of enemata. This small sophisticated pump became widely used throughout Europe and John Weiss was hailed by many as the inventor of the stomach pump. Unfortunately a major brouhaha ensued as each individual involved declared himself to be the sole inventor and claimed primacy for the discovery.

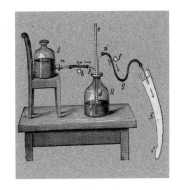

Thomas Alcock in the *Lancet* in 1823 criticized Sir Astley Cooper for his apparent ignorance of the history of the subject: "the comments made by the learned and able Professor, whose approbation is so warmly expressed must be inaccurate or erroneous". Alcock pointed out the contributions of Boerhaave of Holland, Dupytren and Renault and Cadet of France, as well as Orfila's masterly summary of the entire subject.

Although gastric tubes and pumps were originally designed for removal of ingested poison it became apparent to physicians that they might be useful in the study of gastric contents. During the late 19th and early 20th century a variety of devices (*above and below*) were developed for the analysis of gastric secretion.

An analysis of the literature of that time permits the following conclusion. John Hunter may be regarded as the inventor of the stomach tube and was certainly the first to make use of it in England. Physick, who had been a pupil of Hunter, first introduced the tube into America and it was probably used about the same time in France by Dupuytren and Renault. The rival claims of priority established in England by Jukes, Bush, Reed and Evans in 1822 and 1823 may be regarded as modifications of a general principle that had been earlier established. The further utility of the tube was little addressed until 1869 when Kussmaul in his classic publication suggested its use in the treatment of gastric dilatation.

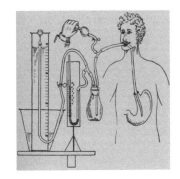

The Contributions of Kussmaul

While previously the use of the stomach tube had been predominantly directed to the removal of poisons, Kussmaul was the first to recognize its advantages under different circumstances. He noted with some regret that in advanced forms of gastric dilatation due to stricture of the pylorus "very exceptionally was it possible to obtain any results in the treatment of this dreadful disease. As a rule it may hardly be possible even to expect an amelioration of the symptoms and never possible to produce a cure".

At the Freiburg Medical Clinic, Kussmaul encountered a 20-year-old young woman, Mary Wiener, who had suffered serious gastric problems for more than a decade, to the extent that she was emaciated, suffered from inanition and continuously vomited to the point that her symptoms could only be relieved by morphine. Kussmaul diagnosed a dilated stomach produced by stricture at the pylorus consequent upon an ulcer, but was powerless to alter the course of the disease. He wrote: "often when I observed the patient in the wretched prodromal stage of vomiting, the thought occurred to me that I might relieve her suffering by the employment of a stomach pump as the removal or large masses of decomposed acid gastric contents

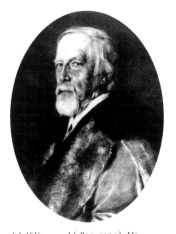

Adolf Kussmaul (1822-1902). His contributions include: being the first to a) treat gastric obstruction with a stomach tube (1867) b) treat gastric ulcer with bismuth (1868), c) attempt esophagoscopy and gastroscopy (1869), d) diagnose mesenteric embolism during life (1867).

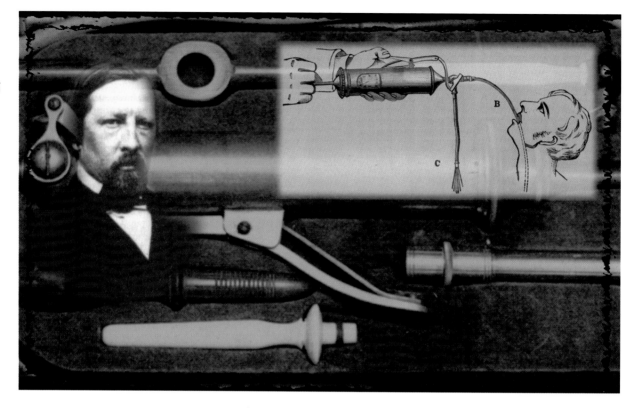

Adolf Kussmaul (1822-1902). Born in Graben near Karlsruhe he practiced as a military surgeon before becoming a peripatetic professor at Heidelberg (1857), Erlangen (1859), Freiburg (1863) and Strasbourg (1876). Possessed of an inquiring mind he was a brilliant scholar and innovative thinker whose contributions ranged from being the first to describe periarteritis nodosa to the description of the peculiar breathing pattern of patients with diabetic coma. On July 22, 1867 he first utilized a stomach pump to decompress the gastric outlet obstruction of Mary Wiener, a young woman with chronic peptic ulcer disease and obstruction. Recognizing that the relief was only temporary he proposed that surgery might be the solution to the problem. By 1869 he had attempted to visualize the interior of the esophagus and stomach but success was precluded by lack of adequate lighting. Towards the end of a life marked by extraordinary medical contributions he wrote poetry under the pseudonym of Dr Oribasius and published a medical autobiography (*Jugendrinnerungen*) detailing his experiences from student to savant.

should cause relief from the agonizing burning and retching at once". Suffice it to say that Kussmaul followed his thoughts and on July 22, 1867 undertook the introduction of the stomach pump. "We withdrew three liters of acid, dirty gray, sarcina containing fluid with particles of food of all kinds undergoing softening and decomposition". Although enthusiastic at this novel treatment, Kussmaul recognized its limitations and particularly in the presence of malignant stenosis of the pylorus, was aware that only relief could be afforded but not cure. He noted with a considerable degree of prescience the possibility that surgery might at some future stage be useful in providing relief for such patients! Such observations may well have generated the impetus that spurred Billroth and his assistants to the consideration of gastrectomy. A further advantage of Kussmaul's early experiments was the renewed interest it created in the utility of the stomach tube for obtaining gastric material. Thus while the therapeutic quotient of his activity was relatively limited, the work of Kussmaul introduced a new era in the development of diagnostic methodology for diseases of the stomach.

DIAGNOSTIC USAGE

It soon became evident that the trauma induced by suction through the stomach tube provided gastric luminal content as well as small portions of gastric mucosa. Gastric syphonage thus became utilized as a tool for evaluating both gastric function and disease.

The invention of rubber allowed Jurgensen to subsequently devise a tube that terminated in a perforated ivory ball and could be guided by a wire stylet into the appropriate site in the stomach necessary for aspiration. A further advance by

Auerbach and Plos provided for the introduction of a double recurrent stomach tube that considerably facilitated gastric lavage. Since the large size of such tubes rendered them somewhat impractical, Hemmeter developed a more useful tube of a smaller diameter that could be advanced further and with less discomfort. In 1874 Ewald utilized a soft rubber tube which could be introduced without the aid of a mandarin and demonstrated that if rubber of a sufficient firmness was used a tube of this type could even be introduced without the use of a rigid component. In fact the actual development of this instrument was serendipitous and supports the old adage that even in medicine chance favors the prepared mind.

Ewald, working at Frerich's clinic, was called to see a patient who had swallowed prussic acid in order to commit suicide. Since no stiff tube was immediately available for gastric intubation, Ewald swiftly acquired a piece of rubber gas tubing from which he removed the sharp front edge and cut two eyelets. After oiling the tube he passed it successfully into the stomach of the unconscious patient and was able to successfully perform the gastric evacuation. Oser of Vienna devised a similar soft rubber tube and by 1871, W. Leube (1842-1911) had concluded that the tube could be used both for therapy as well as a diagnostic tool.

In 1883, Leube established the test meal as a modality by which the motor activity of the stomach could be measured. He demonstrated that a normal stomach emptied within seven hours and went on to further analyze gastric secretion obtained through the stomach tube. Further studies both by himself and F. Riegel (1843-1898) focused on the effect of various chemicals and thermic stimulation in the assessment of gastric secretion. His use of the subsequently much hallowed test dinner of "soup, beef steak, bread and mash potatoes" allowed him to establish that the most favorable time for the removal of the test meal was at the height of digestion. Thus 50 years after the original contributions of William Beaumont (1785-1853) to the physiology of digestion, Leube was able to further amplify the *in vivo* conditions related to the normal physiology of gastric digestion without recourse to the use of a gastric fistula. Of particular interest was his recognition that hydrochloric acid was absent not only from the stomach of patients with gastric cancer but other conditions such as gastritis.

The further study of the nature of acid in the stomach was undertaken by Ewald and Boas in their seminal work "*Physiology and Pathology of Digestion*" (1885-1886). They noted the presence of free hydrochloric and lactic acid in the gastric contents obtained via the tube and com-

The establishment of Gastroenterology as a discipline was due to the contributions and efforts of Ismar Boas (1858-1938) (*left*), Wilhelm Leube (1842-1911) (*center*) and Carl Ewald (1845-1915) (*right*) of Germany. Leube in 1875 intubated the stomach and explored the nature of digestion by developing a "test breakfast." In 1883 Ewald established the rate of gastric emptying and in 1886 his pupil, Boas founded in Berlin the first polyclinic devoted entirely to the study and treatment of gastro-intestinal diseases. Their various texts on the subject of gastric physiology and disease were regarded as the definitive works on the subject until the advent of the Third Reich, when Boas was expelled.

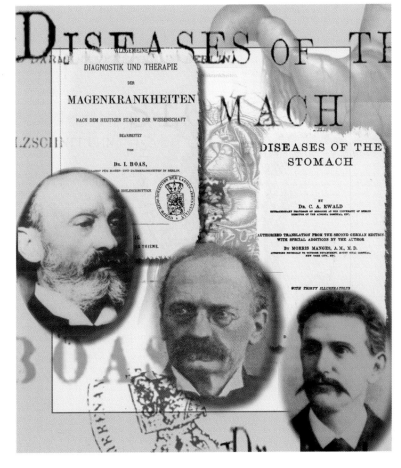

mented on the factors associated with the chemistry of digestion. Ewald subsequently developed the test breakfast and discussed its application in the diagnosis of gastric disease in detail. Further observations dealt with the "expression" method of obtaining gastric juice and the relative advantages of the sampling technique.

DUODENAL EVALUATION

Having successfully traversed the esophagus and initially focused on the stomach, the assessment of the duodenum now became a source of considerable interest. In 1889, Boas managed by judicious manipulation of the gastric tube and massage of the right upper abdomen to obtain duodenal contents from fasting patients whose empty stomach could be kneaded with relatively less discomfort. A similar creative maneuver was undertaken by Boldyreff, who administered a fatty meal that resulted in regurgitation of bile and duodenal contents into the stomach where upon the duodenal secretions were acquired by gastric aspiration.

In 1896, Hemmeter of Baltimore was probably the first to actually instrumentally intubate the duodenum, although L. Turck (1810-1868) had claimed this honor by utilizing his so called "gyromele". This device was primarily intended to outline the boundaries of the stomach by the additional use of palpation over the abdominal area. Hemmeter passed a balloon into the stomach that once inflated allowed a rubber tube to be inserted over a groove on its upper surface and then guided into the duodenum. Unfortunately this methodology proved to be difficult, uncomfortable and impractical. In 1909 Einhorn and Gross developed a tube design (subsequently modified by Rehfuss) that could be used for duodenal intubation. These devices were somewhat similar and consisted of small soft tubes with their tips weighted to facilitate gravity-aided peristaltic passage into the duodenum.

Lyon undertook a further elaboration of the usage of the duodenal tube in 1917 and developed non-surgical biliary drainage by means of a duodenal tube

In 1921, A. Levin of the Touro Infirmary of New Orleans provided a further tube modification that consisted of a smooth rubber catheter without a metal tip that could be introduced via the nostril through the stomach and into the duodenum. Such tubes became widely utilized for the study of gastric contents and fractional gastric analysis was rendered possible in this fashion. Indeed the subsequent studies of gastric function that allowed for the delineation of the action of histamine and gastrin were all predicated on the development of complex multilumen tubes that allowed for not only gastric analysis but also its separation from contamination by alkaline duodenal secretion. Levin worked at the Touro Infirmary (*inset*) established by Moses Touro, whose father had founded the first temple in the USA at Newport, R.I.

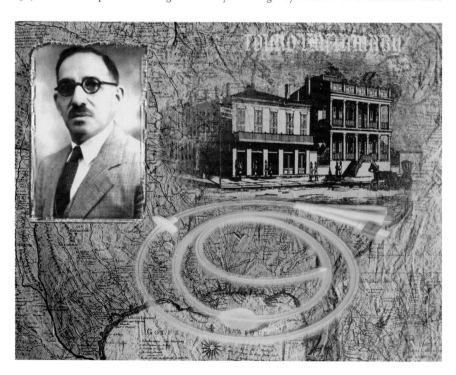

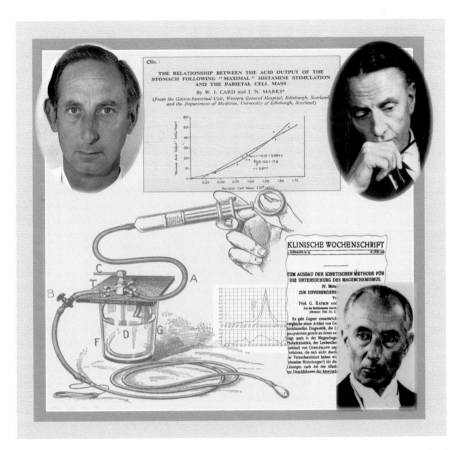

The utility of the "blind tube" was epitomized by its application to the elucidation of gastric secretory function. Gerhard Katsch of Greifswald (1887-1961) (*bottom right*) introduced quantitative gastric function tests (1925) with caffeine or histamine (*kinetic method*) to evaluate gastric secretory capacity. By 1960 I.N. Marks (*top left*) of Cape Town and W. Card (*top right*) working in Edinburgh had successfully defined the relationship of the parietal cell mass to the acid secretory capacity of the stomach. Such studies led to the quixotic proposal that surgery for peptic ulcer disease might be tailored to the acid secretory capacity of an individual patient.

inserted after administration of a solution of magnesium sulfate. In a reversal of strategy, the duodenal tube thereafter also became utilized as a therapeutic device in an intestinal obstruction or ileus, whereby gastric dilatation could be minimized and intestinal secretions aspirated for therapeutic purposes. Thus tubes designed to enter the stomach and the duodenum became standard measures in the evolving area of both diagnosis and therapy pertinent to the management of gastrointestinal disease. The subsequent evolution of such "blind" tubes allowed for the development of the "seeing" tubes. In this respect the initial contributions of Kussmaul in 1868 to the area of esophagoscopy laid the foundations of the concepts that were thereafter amplified and extended by the technical applications of Mikulicz, Rosenheim (1895), Rewidzoff (1899) and, in 1900, G. Kelling (1866-1912). The further elaboration and application of such devices by Chevalier Jackson of Philadelphia (1865-1958) in 1907 and Sussmann of Berlin in 1911 were subsequently overtaken by the unique developments instituted by Schindler and Wolf in 1922. Thus in a relatively short period of time the feather and finger had been replaced by the blind tube and then supplanted by flexibility and finally focus. The story of the seeing tubes is worthy of further detailed consideration since within it lies the genius wrought not only by the vision of great minds and the ingenuity of technology, but a triumph of the melding of clinical application and scientific method.

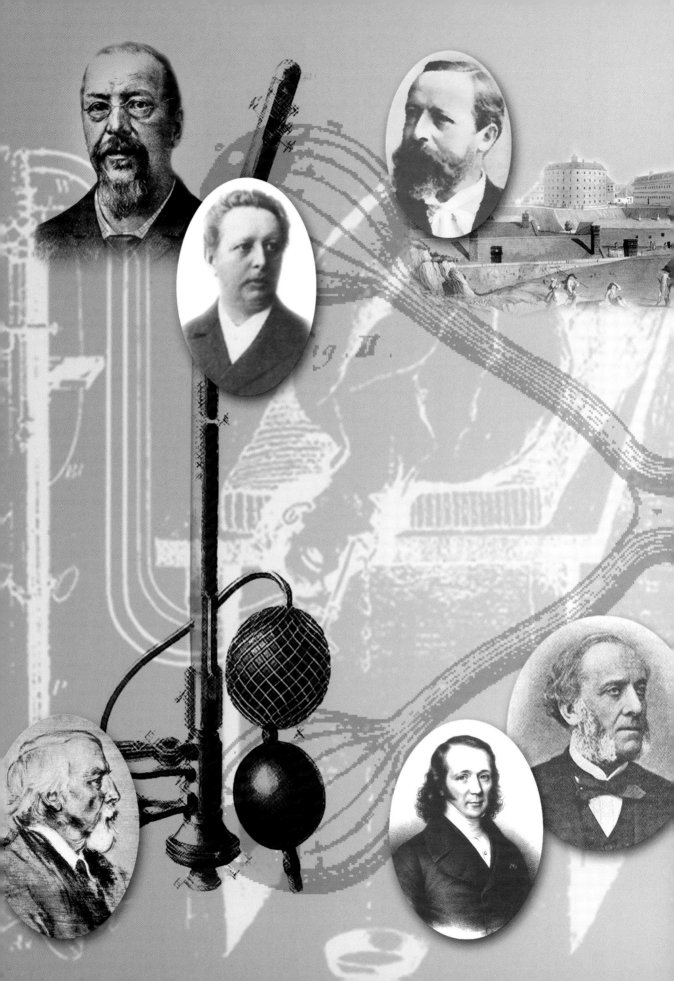

The Evolution of Diagnostic Instruments

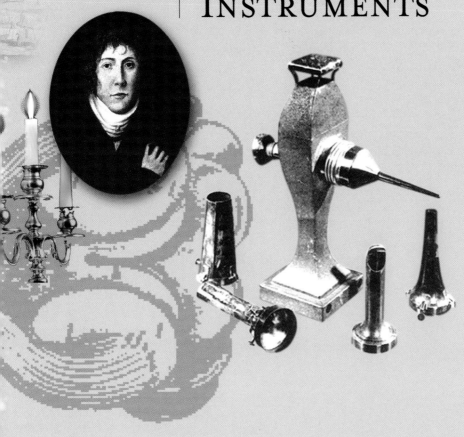

CHAPTER I | *Bozzini and the Bladder*

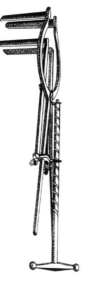

The timeless technical perfection of the speculum found in the ruins of the *"House of the Surgeon"* in Pompeii (c. ACE 80) attests to the ingenuity of the early physicians who sought to explore the dark cavities of the body.

In a world lit only by sun, fire and lunar emanations the critical limitation of early endoscopic devices was the provision of adequate illumination.

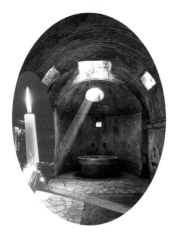

INTRODUCTION

The recognition that tubes were required to gain access to the interior of the body had led to the use of considerable ingenuity to devise safe methods for insertion of such apparatus. It was however evident that the critical limitation in the exploration of internal disease was the paucity of adequate illumination. In this respect the absence of viable light sources was therefore to determine the early development of endoscopic diagnosis and therapy. Under such circumstances it was predictable that since the urethra offered the shortest (and in females the most direct) access to the interior, the earliest target of physicians would become the bladder. Thus gastrointestinal endoscopy would initially lag behind urology as the limits of lighting and the unavailability of instruments capable of adequate flexion around the curvatures of the bowel hampered passage to both the upper and lower reaches of the gut.

The evolution of the instrumentation used in the assessment of the gastrointestinal tract may be regarded as having passed through a number of phases of which each is represented by the dominant instrument form of its time. While it is difficult to precisely delineate the time periods it may be broadly accepted that a "rigid instrument" phase lasted from 1805-1932. This was followed by a Schindler or "semi-flexible endoscope" period (1932-1957) and thereafter the era of "fiber optic endoscopy" was introduced by the work of Hirschowitz. We currently live within the fourth hybrid phase that is an amalgam of video endoscopy, endoscopic ultrasonography and laser Doppler and may probably best be referred to as the technological matrix endoscopy era or the "biovisibility phase" of endoscopic development.

In brief, endoscopy may be regarded as having eventuated with the first attempts of Adolf Kussmaul at gastroscopy in 1868. His work was to a certain extent based upon the Bozzini *Lichtleiter* (1805) and the Desormeux endoscope of 1853. Advances in cystoscopic development by Nitze and Leiter in the 1870s proved seminal in initiating the development of similar instruments for the gastrointestinal tract. Mikulicz in 1881 provided the nexus of endoscopic development within the 19th century by developing a unifying concept that embraced the three critical components of the gastroscope-namely an electric light source, an optical system and a tubular endoscope body. The early part of the 20th century was dominated by rigid endoscopes of which the H. Elsner (1911) and the Schindler (1922) gastroscope were the best accepted. In 1932 the introduction by Schindler and Wolf of the semi-flexible endoscope revolutionized gastroenterology and remained the epitome of instrument design until the introduction of fiber optic instruments by B. Hirschowitz in 1957. Within a decade of this extraordinary innovation, endoscopy had escalated from an art practiced with skill, to a discipline that by the end of the 20th century would successfully embrace the new horizons of biotechnology.

UROLOGICAL ENDOSCOPY

The initial attempt to visual the inside of the bladder cavity was undertaken by Philip Bozzini (1773-1809) of Frankfurt am Main who in 1806 described his light conductor or *Lichtleiter*. A round window in the *Lichtleiter* was divided vertically and the aperture fitted to the open end of a urethro-speculum. Since only one half contained the light source (a candle) the urethra could then be viewed through the other half. Unfortunately Bozzini fell prey to the political jealousies prevalent within the faculty of medicine of Vienna and particularly the disdain of J. Stifft (1760-1839) and as a result failed to gain their support. Although the Academicians of the Josephinum perceived some promise in the device, their report concluded that the lighting was insufficient, the area that could be visualized too small and that the instrument itself would be too painful and dangerous to allow for clinical application. This response was in accordance with the age old Sufi concept that for a new idea to be proved correct a hundred wise men must initially reject it!

PHILIP BOZZINI OF FRANKFURT

Prior to 1805 when P. Bozzini first described his light conductor, the interior of the body could only be dimly perceived through orifices and by the use of crude specula and candlelight. While such instruments were of utility the limitations of the illumination hindered their use except in relatively superficial areas such as the mouth, nose, ear, rectum and vagina.

The endoscope developed (1803-1808) by Bozzini was referred to by him as a *Lichtleiter* since he perceived the critical issue to be the need to "conduct light" to the viewed object. The concept of bringing the image to the eye would not be addressed until years later. The endoscope consisted of a vase-shaped housing that contained the light source; a candle and a series of specula each designed for viewing of a specific orifice. While primacy must be accorded to Bozzini for the development of this ingenious device it never achieved practical usage due both to design flaws and the internecine medical rivalry so prevalent in early 19th century Vienna. The premature demise of Bozzini from typhoid in 1809 brought an early and unhappy closure to the first chapter of endoscopy.

Although the Bozzini design may be regarded as having failed, the principles that he had incorporated within the design established the precedents that would be followed by successors. Thus the triad of a light source, a reflective surface and a graduated series of specula formed the basis for next generation of endoscopes conceived by Segalas of Paris and Fisher of Boston.

The first successful endoscope (*Lichtleiter*) was designed by Philip Bozzini (1773-1809) (*top right*) of Frankfurt in 1805. The ingenuity and skill of the design are reflected in the detailed structural design blueprints and provide a thought-provoking legacy to the subsequent evolution of endoscopic design. The original *Lichtleiter* (*bottom right*) is preserved in the American College of Surgeons museum in Chicago.

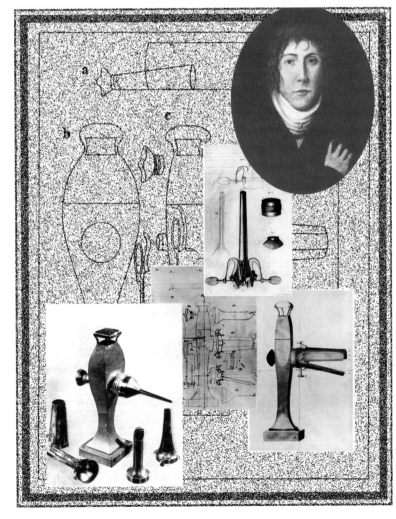

PIERRE SEGALAS (1792-1875) OF PARIS

Two decades later Pierre Segalas (below) demonstrated his own version of the urethro-cystic speculum to the French Academy of Sciences. The endoscope was designed for the purpose of visualizing the interior of the bladder and urethra as well as for the express purpose of crushing bladder stones under direct vision. In 1826 he demonstrated this device (speculum urethro-cystique) to the luminaries of the Academie des Sciences, Paris, and claimed that such was the visual acuity of his device that the smallest print could be read at a distance of 15 inches "in even the most obscure place." This apparatus was designed to view both the urethra and bladder and consisted of two silver cylindrical tubes with open ends, two metal mirrors, two small candles, and a gum elastic catheter. The outer tube had a polished interior and was constructed to be of varying sizing according to the circumstances for which it would be utilized. The second tube was four or five inches long with a bore of equal to but never greater than the first tube, blackened inside and designed to shade the eye from all extraneous light. Light was projected along tubes by means of two conical mirrors between which the two candles were placed.

Segalas used his speculum chiefly for urethroscopy and was able to identify both granulating ulcers as well as strictures. In addition to utilizing it for diagnostic purposes, he applied cautery to the mucosa and also undertook further examination of the bladder. He reported: "in a three-year-old girl, a silver sound proved the presence of a large calculus and examination with the urethrocystic speculum led me to believe it was composed of calcium phosphate, that is to say very friable, which enabled me to use lithotrity for its removal."

Pierre Segalas (1792-1875) of Paris (*top right*) and a model of the design of his urethro-cystic speculum (*top left*). The numerous hospitals of Paris (*borders*) and their eminent physicians vied bitterly for primacy in the introduction of novel and innovative therapeutic devices and techniques. The use of this instrument was relatively simple. Initially the urethral tube was introduced over a gum elastic catheter as far as the obstruction and the catheter thereafter withdrawn. The ocular tube was then placed in line with the first tube in order to set it in the central part of the cone reflector. Simultaneously two lighted candles were held in front of the base of the cone on either side of the ocular tube. The eye could then be applied to the eyepiece and the direction of the apparatus varied according to the part of the urethra or foreign body one being observed.

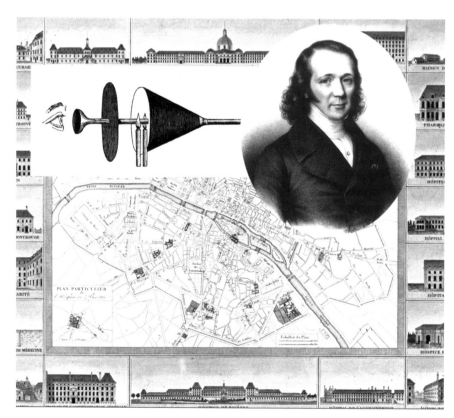

Such was the impact of the demonstration that it instigated a Gallic conflagration as the doyens of Parisian surgery including A. Nelaton (1807-1873), Gabriel Guillon and Baron C. Heurteloup (1793-1864), rose in arms each proclaiming their own undeniable primacy in the field. As with all novel devices rival claimants soon sought to share credit. In a letter to the Academie des Sciences in 1827 Heurteloup bitterly protested the duplicity of Segalas. He stated: "knowing that I had lodged with the Secretariat of the Institute, drawings of an apparatus for viewing the inside of the bladder by means of "lampyres," commonly called glow worms, M. Segalas hastily constructed a reflecting apparatus, which he presented to the Academie as being suitable for this purpose but without admitting that I was the originator of the idea." Six years later Gabrielle Guillon in 1833 demonstrated a *speculum uretri* designed on the same principle as that of Segalas but somewhat simpler to use. In 1850 Nelaton used an endoscope of similar type but without much reported success.

John Fisher (1797-1850) of Boston

Although much of the early progress in endoscopy emanated from Europe, John Fisher of Boston in America was an early contributor to the subject. In 1827 J. Fisher, aware of the work of Bozzini and Segalas, described a similar endoscopic apparatus using a candle, reflective mirrors and a tubular speculum. His principal innovation was the inclusion of a double convex lens to amplify the image. Fisher claimed to have originally designed this endoscope while a medical student in 1824, to visualize the cervix of a woman patient whose modesty forbade his close examination. He recounted that his motivation in this task reflected his "strong and chivalrous desire to protect her feelings of delicacy". Isaac Hayes writing in The Philadelphia Journal of the Medical and Physical Sciences (1827) commented upon the work of Fisher and noted the probable primacy of Messieurs "Bombolzini" and Segalas and hinted darkly at the improbability of such instruments in their current form being of any clinical utility. Of interest in this article was the prescient comment that reflected a quote by Prof. R.M. Patterson who had suggested the possible use of "galvanism" as a means whereby such "dark cavities" might be better illuminated!

Antonin J. Desormeaux (1815-1881) of Paris

As a surgeon particularly interested in urological problems Desormeaux was well aware of the urgent need for access to the urethra and bladder. His work in this area began in 1852 and was presented to the Academie des Sciences, Paris on November 29, 1853 where it was received with acclamation. Secure in his accomplishments Desormeaux credited Segalas with primacy and acknowledged his support in the design process. Although he initially considered the use of electricity for the light source Desormeaux rejected this consideration stating "it is too cumbersome to be carried around and requires an assistant" (to regulate the batteries). Displaying true and formidable Gallic *savoir faire* he also noted "It would moreover

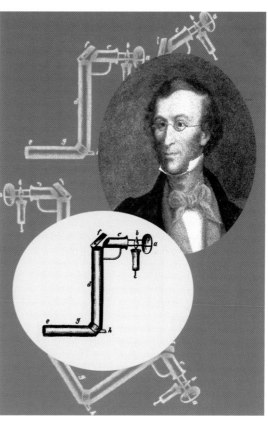

John Fisher (1797-1850) (*top right*) claimed that the need to preserve the modest of a prim Boston matron provided the initial impetus to develop a cystoscope. The Fisher cystoscope (*bottom left*) was comprised as follows. Light was projected through the tube onto a mirror (F) that reflected it onto another mirror (G) by which it was directed along the tube into the cavity. The illuminated field could then be viewed through a window in the mirror (F). Although a system of lenses was added to sharpen the image, the light provided under these circumstances was poor. A modification subsequently introduced by Professor Paterson to amplify the light by use of the Drummond light or electric light was not successful. In his description of this apparatus, Fisher noted that "Bombolgini" of Italy had in 1827 described an endoscope for the inspection of the stomach, uterus, and bladder, but regretted that this important reference could not be identified.

double the price of the instrument!" Instead he therefore chose to use a lamp fueled by mixture of alcohol and turpentine (gazogene) for illumination. As a result of his promotion in 1862 to chief surgeon at the Necker hospital in Paris, Desormeaux was able to widely popularize his endoscope in the treatment of urological disease and his monograph *"De l'Endoscopie"*, published in 1865, played a significant role in the popularization of endoscopy.

Antonin Desormeaux (1815-1881) of Paris (*top*) was responsible for the introduction of the first effective endoscope (*bottom*) and his painted illustrations (*right*) provided critical and novel documentation of pathology. Prior to his contributions the future of endoscopy appeared to have been relegated to obscurity by the use of clumsy and unacceptable instruments. In 1853 he demonstrated to the Academie de Medecin a method whereby he could adequately light deep cavities. This was accomplished by the use of a lamp with a bright flame produced by a mixture of alcohol and turpentine placed between the reflector and the lenses. The latter focussed the light on a flat mirror that reflected it along the catheter so that the surgeon was able to view the illuminated field via an opening in the center of the mirror. A straight sheath with a lateral fenestra served for urethroscopy and for the bladder he used a coude sheath with a glass fenestra close to its end. The publication in 1865 of his magnificent text (*right*) on the subject, *"Traitë de L'Endoscopie"*, was the culmination of the two decades that he had spent in establishing endoscopy as a viable entity.

In addition to his contributions to diagnostic endoscopy Desormeaux developed endoscopic urethrotomy (under direct vision) utilizing a thin knife with a terminal button as well as becoming first to excise a papilloma of the urethra.

Background courtesy of Le Musée d'Histoire de la Médicine, Paris

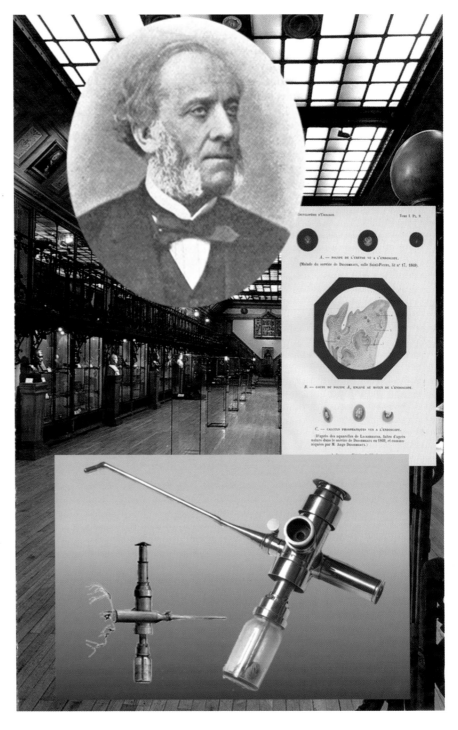

Such was the widespread acceptance of the work of the Parisian that by 1870 the Transactions of the Medical Society of the State of New York carried a report from Robert Newman that strongly supported the use of endoscopy in the management of diseases of the female bladder and urethra. Newman was particularly concerned that endoscopic success could be marred by the use of poor quality instruments and abjured his colleagues from criticism of the technique if a sub-optimal outcome reflected the utilization of shoddy devices. This broadside aimed at instrument makers was somewhat unfair since a number of reputable American instrument makers including J.H. Gemrig (Philadelphia) and G. Tiemann & Co. (New York) were by the 1870s already seriously involved in high quality endoscope manufacture. Indeed the Desormeaux endoscope at a price of $150 was the second most expensive item in the entire Tiemann American Armamentarium Chirugicum catalogue of the time.

FRANCIS CRUISE (1834–1912) OF DUBLIN

Francis Cruise of Dublin described a more successful instrument in 1865. This device was quite similar to that of Desormeaux and produced a more intense light since the lamp was fueled by a mixture of camphor and petrol. The bladder was lighted and viewed through the glass end of the tube introduced along a coude sheath.

Sir Francis Richard Cruise (1834–1912) of Dublin (*bottom left*) studied at Trinity, learnt to shoot in Connecticut, became a splendid cellist, was appointed honorary physician to King Edward VII and knighted by Queen Victoria. He believed in "the direct exploration of organs for the elucidation of their physiology and pathology" and having graciously acknowledged the contributions of Desormeux sought actively to improve the illumination of his device by redesigning the lens and lamp system (*top right*). His original instrument (*bottom right*) as well as a number of other developmental endoscopic devices (*top left*) may be viewed at the Royal College of Surgeons of Ireland, Dublin (*background*).

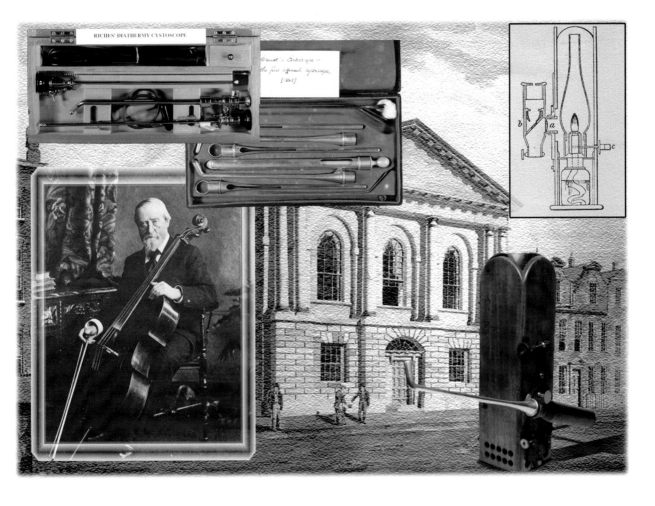

Among the earliest of endoscopic instruments to include optical systems were those designed by the French engineer Gustav Trouvé (*top left*) who in 1870 constructed a polyscope (*top right*) used mostly for laryngeal observations. The most critical feature of the Trouvé polyscope was the improvement that had been made to the intensity of lighting and the stability of the electrical supply (*center*). This allowed a far brighter and uniform visual appreciation of the body cavity. Unfortunately there is little evidence that this device was much used to study the stomach. It is noteworthy that Josef Leiter and Johann von Mikulicz of Vienna subsequently adopted the lighting principles initially developed by Trouvé. Although the electric platinum loop lamp had been introduced in 1845 it had not been satisfactory for endoscopic usage before 1867. Thus the invention of the incandescent lamp by Edison in 1879 provided a much-awaited solution to the critical problem of illumination that had plagued the early endoscopists.

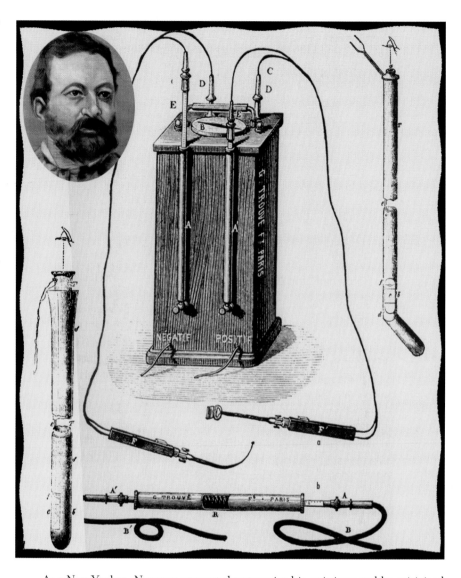

Opposite page
The urologist Max Nitze (1848-1906) (*right*) and Fritz Leiter (*top*), an instrument maker of Vienna, together designed and produced the first effective cystoscope. Their collaboration dissolved after acrimonious disagreements in regard to the optimal design for a gastroscope. With the departure of Nitze to a position in Berlin, Leiter collaborated with Mikulicz in the development of endoscopes for the esophagus and stomach.

As a New Yorker, Newman was not slow to voice his opinions and he criticized the contributions of Cruise of Dublin, Ireland who had sought to improve the illumination of the Desormeaux instrument. Concerned at the low quality illumination and the amount of heat generated by the gazogene lamp, Cruise had substituted a paraffin lamp. Although this modification produced a far brighter light it generated considerable heat and as a result Cruise was forced to house the lamp in a large wooden box for insulation. Newman decried this alteration of the Desormeaux endoscope and declared the instrument as reconfigured by Cruise as "almost too clumsy for manipulation."

In 1867, E. Andrews of Chicago attempted to improve the Cruise endoscope by using a burning magnesium wire but achieved little success. In the same year, in Europe, Julius Bruck (1840-1871) of Breslau and Milliot of Paris using a concept derived from galvano-cautery, independently had the idea of using a loop of platinum wire as an electrical filament. While this device yielded an extremely bright light, it emitted intense heat, required a considerable amount of electricity and the use of a cooling system. To obviate these problems modifications of the system were devised initially by a Parisian engineer Gustav Trouvé. Trouvé in fact went on to design a wide variety of electrical and scientific instruments of which the "polyscope" (introduced in 1870) would become the best known.

Although the Desormeaux endoscope was widely used throughout the United States and Europe, the value of cystoscopy was regarded as modest since most conditions such as bladder tumors were beyond the scope of successful surgery at that time. In 1867 Julius Brück of Breslau designed an unusual instrument, the *diaphanoscope*. This technique involved the introduction of a lamp lit by electric current and cooled by water into the rectum. A speculum was then inserted into the bladder and the interior of the bladder inspected via the transmitted light. This technique was adopted by contemporary gastroenterologists who after filling the stomach with water introduced a light into the cavity. This enabled inspection through the anterior abdominal wall (if sufficiently thin) of the front of the stomach and masses were evident as shadows.

Max Nitze - A Workable Cystoscope

Credit for the development of the first effective endoscope resides with Max Nitze (1848-1906). In March 1877 he constructed an instrument which incorporated the newly described incandescent platinum wire lamp, cooled by water at the end of the cystoscope. Although excellent vision could be obtained, the direct vision telescope provided only a limited field of vision and the heat generated by the platinum wire caused some difficulty. Understanding the need for better technical support in developing his concepts, Nitze collaborated with Leiter, an instrument maker in Vienna.

As a result of their work the Nitze-Leiter cystoscope (*right*) was produced in 1879 and although functional, was difficult to use given problems with its light-

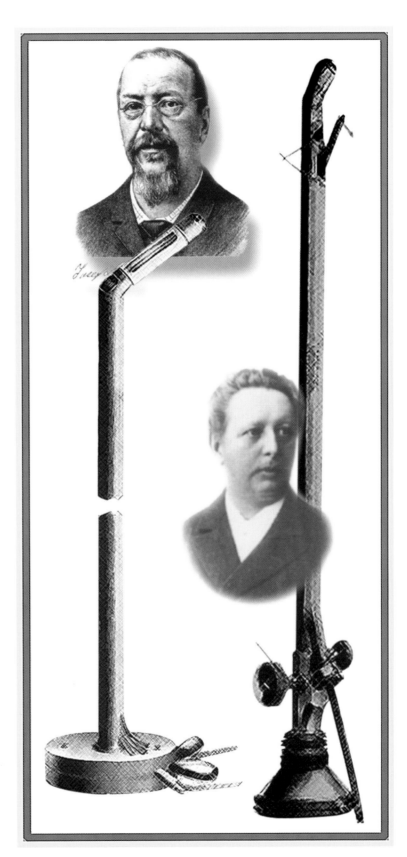

ing and cooling systems. One year later in 1880, the Edison incandescent lamp became available and David Newman of Glasgow in 1883 was the first to incorporate it into a cystoscope. Unfortunately the electric endoscope of Newman was not particularly effective and its relatively large size and clumsiness confined its usage to the female bladder. It consisted of a terminal glass window on the end of a conical tube protected by a tip that could, after introduction, be moved aside by the use of a lever. The electric lamp was then introduced in the bladder separately, as were ureteric catheters. Leiter, however, persisted with the further development of electrical instruments and in 1886 successfully incorporated the Edison lamp into a cystoscope constructed for von Dittel. A year later Nitze recognizing the virtue of this light followed suit.

Joaquin Albarran (1860-1912) (*right*), born at Sagua la Grande, Cuba, was the pupil of the acclaimed Parisian professor of genito-urinary surgery Felix Guyon (1831-1920), originally from the island of Reunion. Having been the gold medallist of the Paris Faculty for two successive years (1888-9) Albarran was appointed *professeur agrégé* in 1892. By 1905 his innovative contributions had revolutionized urological surgery and he had become one of the most acclaimed teachers of the faculty. His design of a moveable lever to facilitate ureteric catheterization (*left*) pre-dated similar devices for cannulation of the duodenal ampulla by more than half a century and was unknown to McCune when he undertook the first successful transduodenal biliary cannulation in 1957.

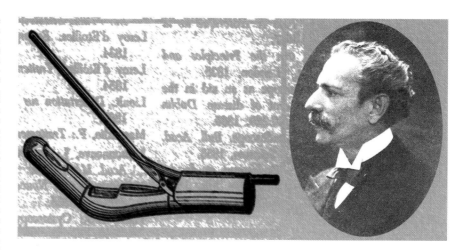

In 1876, Joseph Grünfeld (1840-1910) was the first to successfully catheterize the ureter under direct vision using a malleable catheter which he introduced into the bladder alongside his glass-ended endoscope. Although it contained a more complex optical system and thus produced a clearer image, illumination was a problem and visibility poor. This procedure was subsequently facilitated in 1897 by J. Albarran's (1860-1912) introduction of a cystoscope with a movable lever to guide the catheter. This innovation facilitated intubation of the ureter and catheterization of the ureters led to an understanding of renal pathology, thus opening the way to the development of kidney surgery. The subsequent extrapolation of this technique led to intubation of the papilla of Vater and the development of therapeutic biliary and pancreatic endoscopy.

Indeed the future development of gastrointestinal endoscopy would to a large extent be presaged by the contributions of the early urological surgeons and to a lesser extent the experience of the obstetricians. Such physicians were often faced with dramatic and common problems such as stone impaction, obstructed labor and bleeding and were perforce required to develop novel solutions that required both access to the interior and the ability to intervene. To Adolf Kussmaul of Freiburg is due the credit for first seeking to introduce to the gastrointestinal tract the principles that had been acquired by urethro cystoscopists.

Gastrointestinal Endoscopy | Chapter 2

Open Tubes and Sword Swallowers

Although the introduction of tubes into the upper gastrointestinal tract may be claimed to predate the contributions of Kussmaul he deserves the credit for the first, albeit unsuccessful attempt at endoscopy of the stomach. Thus, in 1868 in Freiburg, Kussmaul utilizing an instrument comprising a straight open tube introduced by aid of an obturator attempted to visualize the gastric lumen. Unfortunately since insufficient illumination was available and the field of vision unsatisfactory the study was discontinued. In Paris at this time, endoscopy of the urethra, urinary bladder and rectum was already well accepted and the endoscope originally described by Desormeaux in 1853 was recognized as being of considerable utility. The Desormeux device had been accepted for use in a number of European countries with some local modifications, and such "endoscopes" were in use even at the clinic of Kussmaul.

Since the esophagus was more difficult to traverse than the urethra, would-be endoscopists of the upper gastrointestinal tract required help both with instrument design and the mode of introduction. They therefore turned to engineers and sword swallowers. Aware of the skill of sword-swallowers, who were able to introduce a straight sword from the mouth to the stomach, physicians interested in endoscopy, such as Cambell of Glasgow and Kussmaul of Germany, enlisted their services in seeking to develop a technique that might be safe for patients.

Kussmaul had since 1865 directed his attention to the problem of access to the stomach and had initiated a renaissance of the gastric tube at the clinic in Freiburg. As an aftermath to the use of "blind" intubation he had already undertaken direct esophagoscopy, using a tube-shaped speculum to which he had attached the endoscope of Desormeaux for illumination. Further information having been obtained after study of a sword-swallower introducing his sword, prompted design modifications of the original instrument that had been utilized for esophagoscopy.

In 1868 A. Kussmaul (*left*) was the first to attempt gastroscopy. The technique he employed to introduce the rigid instrument was based upon that practiced by sword swallowers (*right*). The device (*bottom*) was based upon that previously used by Desormeaux of Paris (1865) to study the bladder. A long, rigid speculum was introduced into the stomach and the proximal tube component attached as the light source. The latter was provided by an attached *gasogen lamp*. Unfortunately the light was inadequate and Kussmaul could not adequately discern detail.

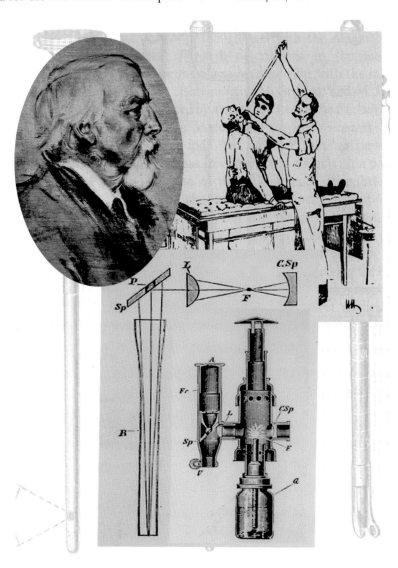

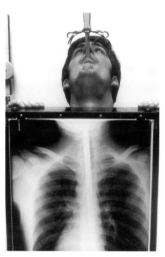

A contemporary 20th century
sword swallower
(Courtesy of Brad Byers).
The sword swallowing
technique of intubation
remained a critical
limitation in the early
development of endoscopy
and required a rare and
special skill possessed by
few patients and physicians.

The Stoerk Esophagoscope.
The chief design flaw
of this instrument was the
inadequate illumination
provided by the meager
light reflected down the
tube by the mirror.
Von Mikulicz was aware of
this problem and agreed to
collaborate with the
instrument maker Josef
Leiter in the production of
a more efficacious device.

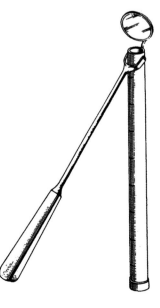

Kussmaul therefore ordered two special tubes each of 47-cm length to be made, one round with a diameter of 13 mm and the other elliptical.

Although the sword-swallower successfully introduced the tube in his usual upright position of performance the examination was unsatisfactory, due to inadequacy of illumination and the copious amount of fluid obstructing the field of visibility. Kussmaul demonstrated the introduction of the tube at the medical section of the *Society of Naturalists* in Freiburg, and even sent his sword-swallower with the tubes for further study at the surgical clinic in Zurich. Although this novel contribution was noted by his contemporaries, Kussmaul did not publish a report and as a result the range of possibilities even with straight instruments, was not recognized until thirty-three years later by Killian (1901).

Despite the contributions of Kussmaul in Freiburg and the innovations of Desormeaux and Trouvé of Paris it would be in Vienna that endoscopy would make its first true steps into the future. The extraordinary milieu of the Allgemeine Krankenhaus, the Josephinum and the intellectual ferment provided by the giants of medicine such as Rokitansky, von Hebra and Skoda enabled the nascent discipline of endoscopy to flourish. Within a relatively brief period Ludwig Turck (the founder of laryngology) and J. Czermak (1828-1873), had introduced the laryngoscope (1858) and subsequently Nitze and Leiter developed the cystoscope (1879). Elements of these designs were incorporated into the construction of the evolving endoscopes of the gastrointestinal tract. As early as 1861 Carl Stoerk (1832-1899) and Friederich Semeleder (1832-1863), former students of Turck, had designed prototype esophagoscopes without much success. Although he persevered for some years Stoerk was never able to persuade his colleagues of the utility of his esophagoscope and brought the issue to the attention of Johann von Mikulicz (1850-1905) the leading pupil and collaborator of Billroth in Vienna.

OPTICAL SYSTEMS AND TUBES

The first endoscopic instruments with optical systems were made by the engineer Trouvé who in 1870 constructed a polyscope (mostly for laryngeal observations) and by the instrument maker Leiter in 1879 who collaborated with Nitze in Vienna to design a cystoscope. The polyscope of Trouvé was not, however, evaluated for stomach endoscopy in human beings. Although the electric platinum loop lamp had been introduced in 1845 its early design flaws precluded endoscopic usage prior to 1867. Thus, the invention of the incandescent lamp by Edison in 1879 provided a much-awaited solution to the critical problem of illumination that had plagued the early endoscopists.

The quotient of the major technical advances that marked the end of the 19th century provided sufficient impetus to enable serious reconsideration of the problem of endoscopy and would culminate in the development of rigid gastroscopy. Indeed within the same year as Edison's discovery (1879), Maximillian Nitze and Josef Leiter constructed the first instrument with an optical system and an electric platinum loop lamp for this purpose and termed it a gastroscope. Unfortunately since Nitze was primarily interested in urology and had already produced a remarkably successful cystoscope, he constructed the gastroscope with an angle at the level of the throat that so restricted the movement of the instrument that it proved to be impractical for use in living subjects. Although Leiter demonstrated this gastroscope to Kussmaul, who had discussed his experience with straight tube-shaped specula with the instrument-maker, the hoped for collaboration failed to eventuate since Freiburg and Vienna were some distance apart.

ESOPHAGOSCOPY AND JOHANN VON MIKULICZ

Johann von Mikulicz was born in Czernovitz in the Bukovina province of the Austro-Hungarian Empire in 1850. By the time of his death in 1905, he had become one of the outstanding surgeons of his time and, were it not for the prominence of his mentor Billroth, would likely have been regarded the preeminent surgeon of the 19th century. Indeed so prolific were his skills that the eponym Mikulicz is associated with at least eighteen diseases, syndromes, anatomical structures, operations, or instruments including chronic hypertrophic enlargement of the salivary and lachrymal glands and the foam cells of rhinoscleroma. Apart from his interest in general disease entities Mikulicz was particularly involved in the surgical management of diseases of the gastrointestinal tract. In his capacity as a close friend and associate of Billroth much of his early experience in this area was gained as a result of the widespread reputation and popularity of the Vienna clinic.

The presence of other medical doyens such as Rokitansky in pathology, Skoda in medicine and J. von Hebra (1847-1902) in dermatology provided considerable impetus for the development of a better understanding of gastrointestinal disease processes and their management. In addition the steady stream of patients with

As an indirect recipient of the largesse of the power of the Austro Hungarian Empire *fin de siecle* Vienna (*map*) and the surgical department of the Vienna medical school proved a fertile field for advances in the diagnosis and management of gastro intestinal disease. Theodor Billroth (*left*) was born on the island of Rügen in the Baltic, trained in Berlin and was professor of surgery in Zurich (1860-67) before accepting the chair in Vienna (1867-94). Although a notable music-critic, accomplished violinist and close friend of J. Brahms, he is best remembered as the pioneer of visceral surgery. Johann von Mikulicz-Radecki (*right*) was Billroth's assistant until 1881 at the Algemeine Krankenhaus in Vienna (*background* with the Narrenturm- Fool's Tower) and thereafter professor at Königsburg (1887) and Breslau (1890). He pioneered the development of esophagogastroscopy, asepsis, advanced gastric and esophageal surgery and wore cotton gloves for a decade prior to the introduction of rubber gloves by Halsted of Baltimore. His eminent trainee E.F Sauerbruch would subsequently deride Schindler, Sternberg and gastroscopy in general as a danger to patients!

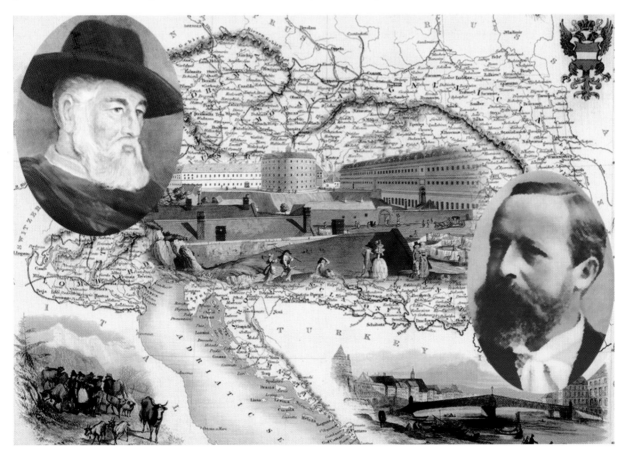

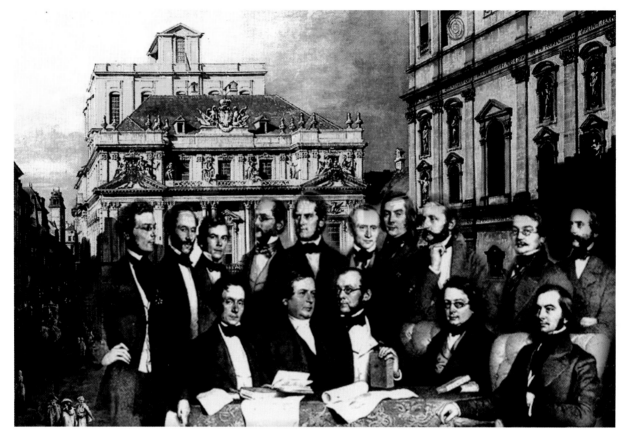

The viviscent intellectual environment of the General Hospital interfaced with the rising power and fervor of Hapsburg Austria facilitated the advance of knowledge in many different areas of clinical endeavor including visceral disease. Over the next 50 years the Vienna medical school would not only train the leaders of European medicine but also set the intellectual pace of progress. The Collegium of the Medical Faculty (*foreground*) of the Vienna University (1853) (*background*) comprised many of the legendary names in medicine. *Back row* (*left to right*): J. Hyrtl, C. Sigmund, J. Unger, C. Haller, E. Brücke, J.R. Oppolzer, T. Helm, F von Hebra, J. Dlauhy. *Front row*: F. Schuh, A. Rosas, C Rokitansky, J. Skoda, and J. Dumreicher.

diverse diseases and the constant presence of brilliant and eager medical minds from throughout Europe provided a fertile environment for the evolution of novel approaches to both diagnosis and therapy. In the midst of such intellectual medical ferment Mikulicz found himself constantly stimulated to explore new territory.

Although Mikulicz was aware of Kussmaul's work and had encountered demonstrations of esophagoscopy he was initially skeptical that the technique would prove to be a viable investigative entity. Thus while he recognized the utility of the procedure he perceived that the limiting issue was the use of reflected light. This belief had been further accentuated by his attendance at a demonstration where Stoerk had failed to adequately demonstrate that mirror reflective light through tubes could be used to illuminate the esophagus. Determined to resolve the conundrum and not dissuaded by the previous attempts, Mikulicz himself thereupon undertook the evaluation of the esophagus in 1880. Recognizing that adequate lighting required collaboration with individuals possessed of different skills to himself, he sought the collaboration of Leiter, the famous instrument maker of Vienna. The expertise of the latter was well known to him since it was none other than Leiter who had in conjunction with Nitze recently succeeded in the development of a practical urethroscope and cystoscope.

Indeed it was the independent (and probably market oriented) belief of Leiter that an instrument designed along similar principles should be developed for the purpose of the visualization of the stomach and the esophagus. Thus Mikulicz and Leiter each for probably different reasons perceived a critical need to develop endoscopic access to the upper gastrointestinal tract.

However, as in all novel endeavors, obstacles abounded. The first problem to be solved involved the possibility of passing a straight rigid tube through the length of the esophagus. Aware, like Kussmaul, of the skills of the sword swallowers in this accomplishment, Mikulicz hired a skilled "swallower" to enable the technique to be studied. In this instance the model was an elderly woman who had developed a remarkable facility for allowing instruments to be passed down her esophagus. Based upon her swallowing skills and the technical expertise of Leiter's assistants rapid progress was made. Thus a finger-thick gum elastic rod was developed that passed without undue difficulty through the esophagus of the experimental subject. Appropriately concerned that the procedure might not be feasible except in individuals specifically trained or possessed of special swallowing abilities, Mikulicz thereafter undertook further experiments on cadavers. In these studies he determined that apart from a slight resistance at the level of the larynx, the only condition necessary to ensure successful esophagoscopy was that the head of the patient be held firmly extended in a sword-swallower's position.

The instrument developed by Mikulicz and Leiter is worthy of comment not only for its primacy in the field but as an early model of the creative and innovative technical development that has characterized the evolution of endoscopy. The esophagoscope exhibited a diameter of 11 to 13mm and was closed by a knob-like head of a stylet or mandarin placed in the lumen of an instrument prior to its usage.

Once the instrument had been successfully introduced to the lower level of the esophagus, the stylet was withdrawn and replaced with a thin flat rod. The rod contained an insulated wiring system and minute conduits utilized for the purpose of cooling. At its proximal end the wire was connected to a Bunsen battery and its terminal end possessed a "u" shaped platinum wire that could be brought to incandescence behind a glass window. The light source or "glow bulb" was then cooled by water that flowed in the tiny circuits surrounding the platinum loop. Since this component of the apparatus only occupied a small space within the tube considerable room was available for visualization of the lumen of the esophagus.

Technique

Having demonstrated that the technique was feasible in trained subjects and having determined the optimal methodology in cadavers, Mikulicz recognized that positioning was of critical importance. Thus the patient was directed to lie on either the right or left side and the esophagoscope with the stylet in place was held like a pen in the right hand of the physician. The base of the patient's tongue was pushed downward and forward by the operator's left index finger and the tube inserted past one corner of the mouth and alongside the finger forwards into the throat as far as possible without discomfort. At this stage the index finger was withdrawn and the instrument itself utilized to keep the tongue depressed. After some uncomfortable experiences using this technique, it became apparent to Mikulicz that morphine in quite substantial doses was necessary to overcome the practical difficulties and dangers associated with gagging and anxiety. A further critical obstacle was the crycopharyngeal sphincter but possessed of considerable skill and patience, Mikulicz recognized after practice that simple application of mild, consistent pressure without undue force soon engendered sphincteric relaxation and passage of the scope into the body of the esophagus. In his initial description of the technique in 1881, Mikulicz emphasized points that are valid to this day and stated that much patience and minimal pressure were critical to avoid damage.

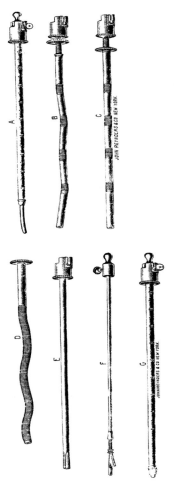

The individual components of the Mikulicz esophagoscope (1881). Attachment of the Leiter panelectroscope (a universal light source for all endoscopic tubes) (bottom) to the proximal end rendered it the first practical and functional esophagoscope.

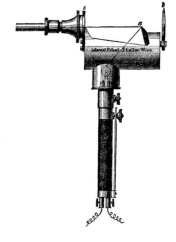

OBSERVATIONS

The clinical observations that Mikulicz provided regarding the esophagus are of considerable interest and attest to his skill and clinical perspicuity. He noted that in a normal organ the mucosa appeared the same throughout, being a uniform pale red traversed intermittently by tiny blood vessels and commented that the smoothness of the mucosa produced a glaring effect that made visualization difficult. This presumably reflected the nature of the light source and was further accentuated by the fact that in the absence of an air insufflation device the walls of the cervical esophagus collapsed around the front of the instrument.

It was Mikulicz's assessment that this closure was not muscular, since he noted there was no evidence of resistance to the advance of the instrument, but more likely due to pressure exerted by surrounding organs particularly the trachea. In contradistinction, however he described the thoracic portion of the esophagus as an open canal with direct visualization of the lumen evident more than 8 to 10 cm ahead of the instrument. In this observation Mikulicz differed from his contemporaries who considered the esophagus to be a closed tube. The difference between the closed cervical esophagus and the open thoracic was felt by Mikulicz to be a reflection of the negative intra-thoracic pressure. In addition to these anatomic comments Mikulicz remarked on some functional aspects and asserted that the walls of the esophagus exhibited at least three different types of movement. Firstly a pulsatile motion that was obviously

Although credit for the introduction of the first effective endoscope and the publication of its utility is due to Max Nitze (1848-1906) (*bottom right*) the instrument maker Joseph Leiter (*top right*) played a role in the development. In March of 1877 they constructed an instrument which incorporated the newly described incandescent platinum wire lamp, cooled by water at the end of the cystoscope. As a result of their work the Nitze-Leiter cystoscope was produced in 1879 and although functional was difficult to use given problems with the lighting and the cooling systems. Although excellent vision could be obtained, the direct vision telescope and the limitations of the lens system (*center*) provided only a limited field of vision. Nevertheless within a short time the apparatus was widely available and could even be transported to different medical facilities (*left*). Subsequent developments included the introduction of photographic devices (*top left*) and the addition of cautery probes for therapeutic intervention.

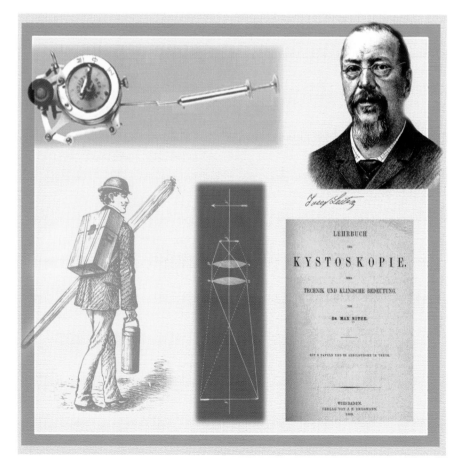

related to the proximity of the heart and the aorta; secondly a respiratory movement and thirdly of particular interest a movement which he rightly recognized as peristaltic. These contractions were not synchronous with the pulse but were associated with swallowing or gagging and could be provoked simply by moving the esophagoscope.

In addition to his sagacious assessment of the physiological nature of the normal esophagus Mikulicz also reported pathological observations and described in detail foreign bodies, cancer, and esophageal compression due to lung disease and aortic aneurysm.

CODA

A fascinating man of considerable technical skill as well as creative brilliance, Mikulicz may well have earned the sobriquet of "the father of esophagoscopy." While he was certainly not the first to attempt esophagoscopy, it is mostly due to his initial efforts that the development of a practical instru-

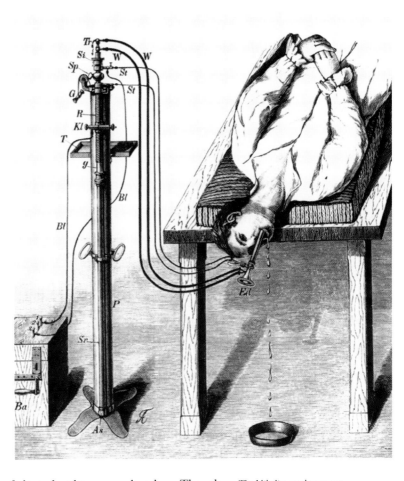

ment capable of furnishing information of clinical utility was undertaken. Though Kussmaul deserves credit for taking the first steps in pursuing the subject of esophagoscopy, there is little doubt that without the subsequent collaboration of Mikulicz and Leiter in Vienna little progress would have been made. Though the development of a safe clinical technique was mandatory, the issue of adequate visualization was a critical element. Thus the introduction of the platinum glow bulb and Leiter's expert technical contributions were paramount in facilitating the progress of Mikulicz. A further propitious factor was provided by the esteemed position of Mikulicz in one of the great surgical departments of the world. Thus information or techniques emanating from the great departments of the Vienna General Hospital (Allgemeine Krankenhaus) were rapidly accorded widespread attention and more often than not accepted as valid.

Furthermore, since Billroth's department was regarded as one of the premier surgical teaching clinics in Europe the numerous visiting physicians soon carried word of the latest advances back to their own cities and countries and thus further amplified the impact of such contributions and novel developments. In this fashion the esophagoscope developed by Mikulicz and the concept of esophagoscopy as a useful clinical tool spread rapidly throughout Europe. Further modifications such as the recognition of the utility of cocaine as a topical anesthetic, the development of suction apparatus and the improvement of the electric light sources resulted in a worldwide rapid amplification of the technique and its widespread usage.

The Mikulicz esophagoscope proved to be of considerable utility and novel information in regard to esophageal conditions was obtained. Its rigidity however required considerable caution during introduction and the extended head position (*right*) was rendered even more incommodious by problems with inadequate pharyngeal anesthesia and excessive salivary secretion. The complex electrical apparatus for lighting (*left*) designed by Leiter was ingenious but cumbersome, in that it required a water cooling system to sustain the platinum lighting elements and a large Bunsen battery to provide power for illumination. Having successfully developed an esophagoscope (1880) and a less effective gastroscope (1881) during his association with Billroth in Vienna, Mikulicz subsequently became the department chairman in Cracow (1882) and then Breslau (1890). These moves and the loss of close contact with Leiter led to a more sustained focus on administration and technical surgery with little further upper gastrointestinal endoscopic development work. Ironically he would perish of a gastric neoplasm in 1905.

EARLY CONSIDERATIONS OF GASTROSCOPY

Recognizing the importance of visual access to the stomach and esophagus, Mikulicz was sensitive to the need to develop effective instruments for this purpose and sought the support of Leiter in this endeavor. The timing was perfect since Leiter and Nitze had quarreled bitterly and Nitze had departed Vienna for Berlin leaving Leiter in possession of a flawed gastroscope and no interested or available clinician to further pursue the subject. Nitze was dissatisfied with the Leiter prototype since he had undertaken experiments in cadavers as well as in living subjects and was of the opinion that the ideal design would comprise an elastic instrument, that could be stiffened during insertion into the patient. The actual instrument produced by Leiter was however analogous to an esophagoscope but possessed a longer elastic segmented component and a side viewing optic window. Nitze considered the experimental version of the gastroscope produced by Leiter as quite inadequate and would neither demonstrate nor publish it and as a result of this personal tension further collaboration became impossible.

Despite this, Leiter demonstrated the instrument at various clinics and in fact vainly attempted to sell this first gastroscope without it having been adequately clinically evaluated. As a consequence of this flawed commercial and quasi-scientific venture subsequent attempts at gastroscope design were poorly regarded.

Frustrated by the lack of progress with Nitze, the obvious flaws of the current instrument and the improbable logistics of working with Kussmaul in distant Freiburg, Leiter reconsidered his position. Thus in 1880 he and Mikulicz undertook to re-evaluate the problem at the General Hospital Clinic in order to develop a more effective design both for the esophagoscope and the gastroscope.

The outcome of their collaboration provided evidence of more thoughtful work and the gastroscope detailed by Mikulicz in 1881 was the first to be based on careful anatomic considerations. As a clinician Mikulicz was particularly concerned with the potential problems posed by introduction and perforation. Dissatisfied with the information gained from the study of sword swallowers he turned his attention to cadaveric experiments in order to determine the most ideal tube type and mode of introduction. In cadavers, a straight tube could be introduced into the thoracic esophagus to the level of the eighth or ninth vertebra, before the convexity of the lower thoracic spine impeded further safe passage. As a result, slightly angled instruments made of hardened rubber were tested, since flexible optical systems were initially considered to be impractical. A further issue of consequence was posed by the need to ensure safe introduction in conscious patients. The use of a vertical position was unsatisfactory due to salivary regurgitation with retching movements, vomiting and discomfort, and it was evident that introduction in the right or left lateral supine position, with the head slightly lowered, was the best. Whether right or left was dependent upon on which of the two instruments were used.

Since introduction of the instrument into a stomach filled with water was difficult and resulted in vomiting, air was preferred. However air insufflated by a stomach tube was eructated during instrument introduction and the stomach could therefore only be inflated with the gastroscope already in position. Examination during mild chloroform narcosis proved unsatisfactory, whereas morphine (0.04 gr.) suppressed the retching and ameliorated pain, rendering examinations of 10-

The Nitze–Leiter Gastroscope, 1879. M. Nitze and J. Leiter constructed the first instrument with an optical system and electric platinum loop-lamp for the express purpose of examining the stomach and termed it a gastroscope. Unfortunately since Nitze was primarily interested in urology and had already produced a remarkably successful cystoscope, he constructed the gastroscope more mindful of urethral rather than cervical angulation. Thus the angulation at the level of the throat proved so pronounced that it restricted the movement of the instrument to the extent that it became impractical for use in living subjects. The abrupt departure for Berlin of Nitze amplified the bitter rift that had arisen between the two collaborators in regard to design flaws and Leiter determined to proceed alone with development of the gastroscope. Despite its obvious clinical shortcomings Leiter thereupon enthusiastically demonstrated the instrument to physicians and vainly attempted to market the first gastroscope without adequate clinical evaluation.

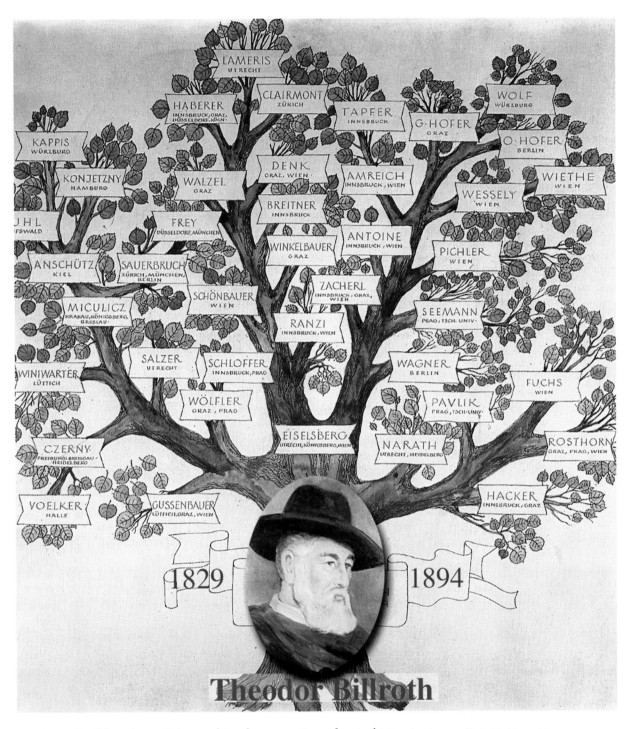

15 minutes feasible and permitting teaching demonstrations of up to thirty minutes.

As a result of his detailed investigations Mikulicz with the aid of Leiter published their final design in 1881. The instrument had a 14mm diameter and was rigid, slightly angled, and possessed both an optical system and a platinum loop lamp cooled by water, as well as a balloon to inflate the stomach with air. A membrane protected the optical system against soiling while the instrument was passed through the esophagus. Since it could only be rotated through 180 degrees, only

Theodor Billroth's surgical dynasty. The family tree of his trainees represents an arbor vitae of the dominant surgical leaders of late 19th century Europe. Many were responsible for innovative developments in visceral surgery and Mikulicz and Czerny in particular contributed to the advance of endoscopy.

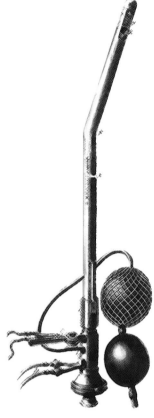

The Mikulicz–Leiter gastroscope 1881. The design was based upon the original Nitze–Leiter cystoscope with a 30° angle in its distal third and a small "mignon" light at the tip. Despite its substantial modifications from the failed Nitze –Leiter gastroscope, Mikulicz was dissatisfied with the device and declined to pursue its further development. Chevalier Jackson with Philadelphian gentility applauded the contributions of Mikulicz, but in so doing damned the device with faint praise by declaring that the instrument had been doomed to failure since the principles of a cystoscope could not be adapted to the stomach, "At the door of the Nitze cystoscope must be laid the blame of the practical failure of gastroscopy up until the present day. The attempt to adapt the cystoscopic principles to the totally different conditions in the stomach resulted in the misdirection of the earnest, able, scientific efforts of Mikulicz, Rosenheim and Rewidzoff."

half the circumference of the stomach could be inspected, and thus two instruments were necessary to examine the entire stomach.

Mikulicz was thus the first to really inspect the stomach with the gastroscope and at the time of his initial report, had examined more than twenty cases wherein he described not only the movements of the pylorus, but also the appearance of gastric ulcers and cancers. In 1896 his collaborator Kelling in a report of 20 patients published the first observations of a carcinoma without any palpable tumor. This report was of considerable significance since such lesions would not have been otherwise diagnosed at that time. Although Kelling increased the efficacy of the gastroscope by adding a rotating optical tip, the modification rendered the instrument difficult to introduce and the examination painful.

Despite having generated considerable progress and immeasurably contributing to the advance of gastroscope design Mikulicz discontinued his gastroscopic endeavors. Although his enthusiasm had diminished because of technical difficulties with the loop lamp and some misadventures with patients, personal events rendered further work in this area difficult. Nevertheless his contributions to the development of the esophagoscope fared far better. Dismissing the curved cystoscopic concept he reverted to the principle of the straight rigid shaft as initially utilized by Kussmaul. Although this design posed difficulties with introduction it enabled direct visualization of the esophagus without the inclusion of a complex system of lenses and prisms and benefited from the inclusion of an incandescent electric light. The latter invention had been described by Edison in 1879 and came to the attention of Leiter in 1883 at the International Electrical Exhibition in Vienna. Swift to foresee its possibilities Leiter initially modified it for cystoscopic usage in 1886 and thereafter reconfigured it for the esophagoscope. The small (mignon) bulb eliminated the need for the platinum loop lamp and abrogated the use of the large and clumsy water cooling system. As a result the Mikulicz esophagoscope became the first instrument of this type which was clinically viable.

Sadly for the science of endoscopy Mikulicz had by this stage reached a level of such seniority and accomplishment in Vienna that he sought to further his career elsewhere. The different professional problems posed by his departure in 1882 initially to the Chair of Surgery at Krakow and thereafter Breslau in 1890 altered the subsequent focus of his endeavors and responsibilities.

ROSENHEIM OF BERLIN

In 1895 the problem was taken up again by Rosenheim who had previously obtained considerable experience with esophagoscopy and had in addition taken the time to study tube introduction in cadavers. He demonstrated that by proper manipulation and experience even straight rigid instruments could be introduced into the stomach in up to 90% of patients and in 1896 published details of a gastroscope of his own design. Although there was little market for his instrument the principles that he utilized were the forerunners of subsequent developments.

The gastroscope that Rosenheim developed was straight, 12mm in diameter, and consisted of three tubes that inserted into each other. This relatively simple appearing device terminated in a straight rubber tip, although in an early version, the tip had been slightly angled to facilitate introduction into the cardia. The outer tube carried a platinum loop lamp with a water-cooling jacket. So critical was this latter feature that after every fifteen seconds of inspection the instrument had to be switched off for cooling. Without the water cooling only ten seconds inspection was possible before over-heating occurred. The middle tube had a window at one side and the inner tube contained an optical system that allowed both anterior and posterior viewing. Rotation of the middle tube permitted closure of the window while the instrument was in the stomach thereby protecting the optic from mucus and fluid.

The day prior to the gastroscopy it was the practice of Rosenheim to introduce a straight metal sound to ensure that the passage to the stomach was free. Although he had performed this procedure on more than 100 occasions his first report documents his successful experience with twenty patients. The abrupt termination of his studies was rumored to have followed an accident and the device languished until Rewidzoff of Moscow in 1897 suggested a modification in making the outer tube flexible. Unfortunately for Rosenheim his contributions were not well received and the instrument was not adopted by his peers with the result that little information pertinent to its usage was ever published.

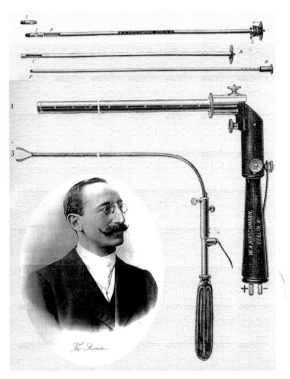

Theodor Rosenheim of Berlin (1895) developed a straight gastroscope 12mm in diameter that consisted of three tubes inserted into each other (top). His adept usage of this device led to considerable clinical success and his published reports confirmed its utility. For reasons that are unclear and rumored to relate to a perforation, the instrument did not achieve popularity and Rosenheim retired from the practice of endoscopy. Other technical innovations introduced by Rosenheim included an esophageal forceps (bottom) and esophagoscope for the removal of foreign bodies.

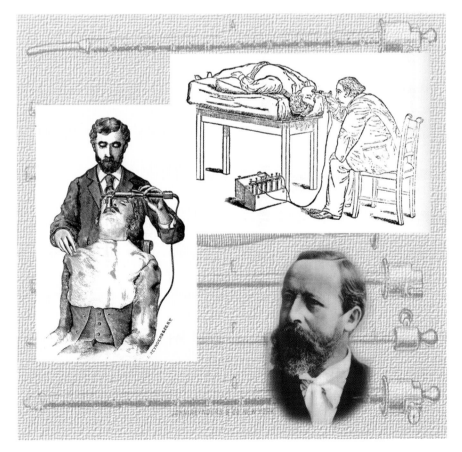

The Mikulicz esophagoscope (1881) and the Leiter pan-electroscope (1887). The further development of the open rigid tube by Mikulicz (bottom right) and Leiter led to the production of an efficient and effective esophagoscope (left). The addition by Leiter of his "pan-electroscope" (right) was critical in resolving the issue of illumination. It provided a battery operated universal light source for all endoscopes and was based upon an Edison lamp that provided illumination by reflecting light from a diminutive electric bulb built into the handle. The resolution of the problem posed by inadequate illumination represented a major advance in endoscopy.

CHAPTER 3 | *From Technology to Vision*

INTRODUCTION

In the three decades after *fin-de-siecle* Vienna a diverse group of physicians, engineers and optical experts from a variety of countries participated in the evolution of the endoscope. While Austria (particularly Vienna) and Germany continued to dominate the development of the science in the early part of the century, World War I hindered progress as resources were diverted to martial matters and physicians inducted into military service. The subsequent advent of Nazi Germany and the Austrian *Anschluss* resulted in the demise or forced immigration of many talented scientists and engineers to America, with the result that the initial impetus provided by European skills was translocated to the New World. Nevertheless the first three decades of the 20th century were times of great flux and numerous individuals participated in the development of exciting designs and instruments as novel technology was transferred to medical applications. Of paramount importance in this context were five areas of innovation: 1) the availability of a power source —electricity, 2) the introduction of an adequate incandescent light source (illumination), 3) advances in pharmacology and anesthesia, 4) the elaboration of physical materials more conducive to the construction of such apparatus and 5) the expansion of the theory of optical systems. The entire concept was, however, most powerfully driven by the physicians of the time who, inspired by the vigor which Boas, Ewald and Leube had devoted to the development of the discipline of gastroenterology, recognized the vital necessity of gaining visual access to their domain of interest.

A considerable impetus to the advance of endoscopy at the turn of the 19th century was provided by progress made in the area of electricity and illumination. Thus sunlight and candlelight augmented by mirrors and lenses were supplanted by first gaslight, and thereafter electrically heated carbon and platinum filaments. In addition unwieldy and clumsy batteries were replaced by more efficient power sources and large lamps supplanted by miniature bulbs suitable for intra-cavity illumination.

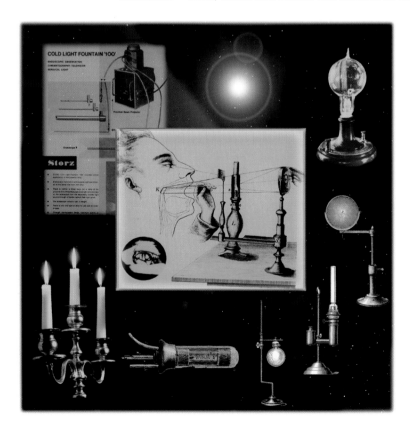

ELECTRICITY

The field of electricity was initiated by the contributions of Gilbert in the 17th century and was amplified and extended at the end of the 18th century by the discoveries of Galvani and the construction of the battery by Volta. Almost half a century later Henry and Faraday extended these Italian observations by co-discovering the principle of electromagnetic induction and thereby engendered the subsequent development of the coil, the dynamo and the transformer.

In 1600, William Gilbert (1540-1603), physician to Elizabeth I of England, published his text "*De Magnete*", which described his studies on the effects of minute quantities of

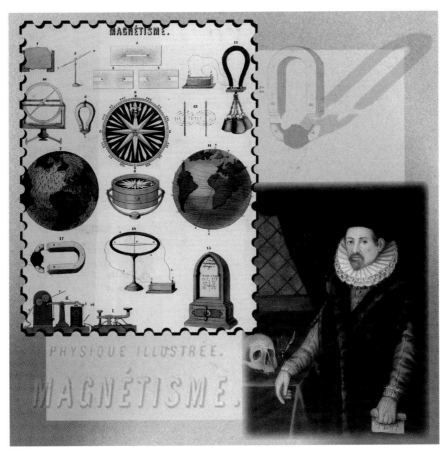

William Gilbert (1540-1603) (*bottom right*), the physician for Elizabeth I of England and an intellect of the Elizabethan age, generated some of the early seminal thought regarding magnetism and provided thoughtful contributions in regard to early concepts of "*electricity*". An enthusiastic proponent of the Copernican hypothesis, he supported the concept that heavily bodies were held in their orbits by a similar agency to that exhibited by lodestones. In 1600 Gilbert published his text "*De Magnete*", which provided the scientific foundation for the subsequent investigation of electricity and magnetism. Thus the lodestone evolved into the compass (*right*) and phenomenology and superstition were supplanted by concepts of electromagnetic waves and invisible particles (*electrons*). Gilbert also studied the effects of minute quantities of static electricity as well as frictional electricity and the electrical properties of amber. He was the first to use the term *electrical* (derived from the Greek word for amber) to apply to the property of attraction arising from the friction of materials such as glass, resin, ceiling wax, sulfur, crystals and amber. His primitive experiments resulted in the production of an electroscope that he called a *versorium*. The discoveries of L. Galvani and the construction of the battery by A. Volta at the end of the 18th century extended the work of Gilbert in the area of electricity. Their work was in turn amplified by the co-discovery almost half a century later by Henry and Faraday of electromagnetic induction (*top right*). The elucidation of this principle led to the invention of the coil, the dynamo, and the transformer.

high-tension electricity, "static electricity" and "frictional electricity," as well as on the electrical properties of amber, glass, resin, sealing wax and crystals. This treatise became instrumental in establishing the scientific foundation of the subsequent investigation of electricity and magnetism. The next important device was the "electrical egg" of the Frenchman, Jean Antoine (Abbe) Nollet, which was achieved by placing a source of high of tension electricity within an evacuated tube. Benjamin Franklin (1706-1790), then resident in France, was captivated by the French preoccupation with electricity and studied the phenomenon with diligence. He demonstrated that lightening was due to an electrical discharge and postulated the "single fluid" theory of electricity in which he coined the terms positive and negative and described electricity as composed of "particles infinitely subtle."

Concomitant with these studies of nature, devices were designed to collect and store large amounts of static electricity. These Kleist or Leyden jars were utilized not only for public demonstrations of the effects of electricity, but for medical treatment and used in attempts to convey electricity through wires.

Prior to the late 18th century, it had been considered that all electrical phenomena could be produced either by friction or atmospheric electricity. However, Luigi Galvani (1737-1798) and Alessandro Volta (1745-1827) of Italy were responsible for the momentous observation that originated when two different conductors were placed in contact with a source of electrical current. The initial experiments of Galvani with "twitching" frog legs suspended by a copper hook to an iron rail had drawn him to the erroneous conclusion of the phenomenon of "animal electricity."

The subsequent demonstration, however, by Volta of the "voltaic pile," a column of alternating plates of silver and zinc or copper and zinc soldered together on one end and separated by moist cloth or leather, confirmed the exogenous source of this electricity. These observations led to the construction of the voltaic cell and raised issues as to whether electricity generated by a voltaic pile was different to that produced by the classic "static" machines.

The most important observation in the evolution of electricity was the identification of the link between electricity and magnetism first proposed in 1820 by the Danish professor, Hans Christen Oersted (1777-1851). Within a year, the French mathematician Andre Marie Ampere (1775-1836) had enunciated the mathematical principle to determine the direction in which the electrical current deviated the needle, and in so doing laid the basis for the study of electrodynamics. This work would subsequently enable George Simon Ohm (1787-1854) to develop the mathematical relationship that embraced current, electrometer force and resistance. In 1831, Michael Faraday (1791-1867) repeated and extended the experiments of Oersted and Ampere, thereby further detailing the nature of the relationship between electrical and magnetic forces.

In addition to his identification of electromagnetic induction, Faraday laid down the principles for the production of continuous induction currents from a coil rotating between magnetic poles. This work led to the identification of the principle of electromagnetic induction and the construction of induction coils and transformers

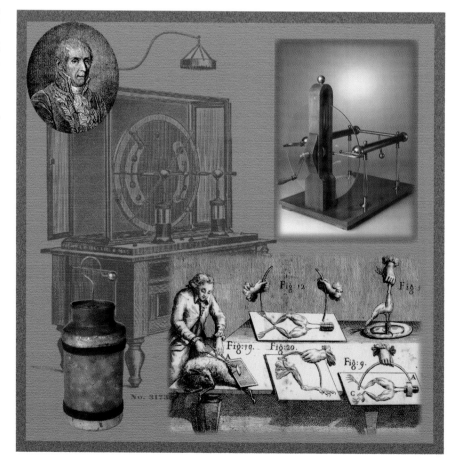

The evolution of electricity from an animal phenomenon to a man made power. L. Galvani's (*top left*) initial experiments with twitching frogs legs suspended by a copper hook to an iron rail had led him to the conclusion of the phenomenon of "animal electricity" (*bottom right*). The subsequent observation of Alessandro Volta that an electrical current originated when two different conductors were placed in contact resulted in a revision of this notion. Although static electricity could be collected in Kleist or Leyden jars (*bottom left*), Volta's demonstration of the "voltaic pile" (a column of alternating plates of silver and zinc or copper and zinc soldered together on one end and separated by moist cloth or leather) confirmed the exogenous source of the electricity. Subsequently electrostatic machines such as those constructed by James Wimshurst (*top right*) were constructed to generate electricity. Further improvements by Wilhelm Holtz (hard rubber plates instead of glass plates covered with tin foil) resulted in devices (*top left*) capable of producing adequate electricity to power either lamps or even generate cathode rays.

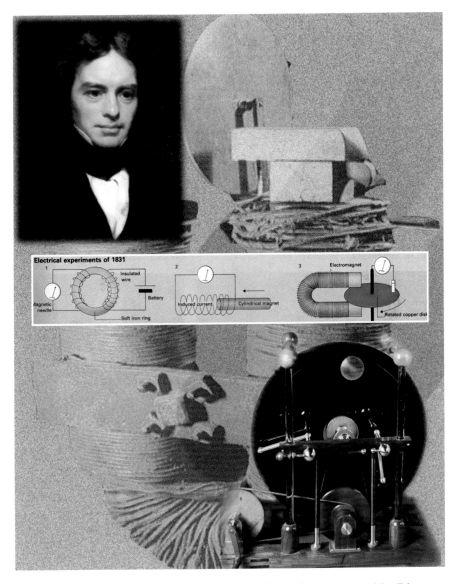

Electrical experiments of 1831

In 1831 the British Scientist, Michael Faraday (*top left*) elucidated the relationship between electrical and magnetic forces. His work moved beyond the electrostatic production of electricity (*right, top and bottom*) and led to the identification of the principle of electromagnetic induction and the construction of induction coils and transformers (*center and left*) adequate to produce electrical currents of high voltage. Heinrich Daniel Ruhmkorff, a Parisian mechanic, utilized Faraday's electro-induction principles to construct an improved induction coil (Ruhmkorff coil) that W.Roentgen utilized to produce X-rays. An additional contribution of Faraday was his recognition that a differential electrical potential applied to two points in an electrolyte resulted in negatively charged particles moving towards the positive terminal, while positively charged ones traveled towards the negative terminal. He designated these charged particles as *ions* (derived from the Greek for travelers) or carriers of electricity and was the first to use the words anode and cathode.

adequate for the generation of the high voltage electrical currents used by Edison to drive his electric lamps. Additionally, Roentgen was subsequently able to utilize such devices in the generation and study of his unnamed X-rays using similar techniques and methodologies. Thus, the energy to adequately illuminate internal aspects of the human body was provided by harnessing the properties of electricity.

THE ROLE OF EDISON

Although light is a vital component of many aspects of life, in few endeavors would it prove to be more critical than in the development of gastroenterology. The subject of illumination thus became both a source and a solution to one of the most critical problem of endoscopy-visibility. A great debt is owed to Thomas Alva Edison (1847-1931), an Ohioan living in New Jersey, whose creative endeavors and inventions allowed him to become regarded as arguably the most prolific inventor in the world. Born in Milan, Ohio, his career as an inventor and physicist would span

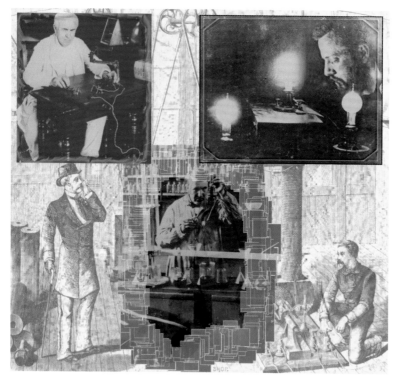

The scientific contributions of Edison in the sphere of electricity and light were rapidly incorporated into the design of endoscopes. During his lifetime Edison generated more than 1,000 patents including the gramophone (1877) and the carbon granule microphone as an improvement of Bell's telephone. Included in his other inventions were a megaphone, the electric valve (1883), the kinescope (1891), a storage battery and Benzyl plants. In 1912, Edison produced the first talking pictures and essentially revolutionized the world of cinematography. In addition to his numerous other contributions, he was the discoverer of thermionic emission previously known as the "Edison Effect." *Top right:* Tessla, whose contributions to the field of electricity amplified those of Edison.

the globe. As a child, following his expulsion from school (he was deemed "retarded"), he became a railroad news-boy on the Grand Trunk Railway and published his own newspaper, the Grand Trunk Herald. During the American Civil War (1861-65) he worked as a telegraph operator and developed an electric vote-recording machine. In 1871, he invented the paper ticker tape and thereafter a "magic repeater" for stock exchange prices. With the proceeds of the sale of these devices he established an industrial research laboratory at Newark, NJ, and in 1876 established himself and his family in close proximity, initially at Menlo Park, NJ, and finally West Orange, NJ, in 1887. By this stage he had amassed enough financial wealth and intellectual influence to provide full scope for his astonishing inventive genius.

The contributions of Edison to endoscopy originated in 1878, when he con-cluded that gas lamps were unreliable, provided an inefficient and ineffective light source and should be replaced by an electric or incandescent light. Within 14 months of this statement, Edison demonstrated 30 different varieties of lamps, each with its own separate switch, which he had created. As a result of this contribution a stable light source became commonplace in the household and workplace and was instantly adapted to a variety of industrial and scientific endeavors. It greatly simpli-fied the light requirements for endoscopic instruments, and was rapidly adopted by a number of experimental endoscopists, including Newman in Glasgow (1883) and Nitze of Vienna soon thereafter.

LENSES AND OPTICS

The phenomena of light and vision have not only fascinated man since the beginning of time, but become an intrinsic part of his exploration of life. The dis-covery of a convex lens made from rock crystal in the ruins of Nimrad provided evi-dence that even the most ancient of civilizations possessed a knowledge of optics. By the end of the first millenium (1000 A.C.E.), the study of the properties of a variety of glass lenses provided the basis for Alhazen to produce a treatise, "*Kitab Al-Manazir*", that dealt with refraction and reflection. This work would form the basis for the sub-sequent development of spectacles, telescopes, microscopes, and eventually the fiber optic endoscopes developed at the end of the second millenium. In 1265, Vitello of Silesia introduced the study of optics into Europe by disseminating and adumbrating upon the original work of Alhazen. The assimilation of this material enabled Savius Aramatus of Pisa (c. 1300) to develop and introduce the concept of spectacles, although such early eyeglasses were cumbersome, being mounted on contraptions of wood, metal or leather. The first application of lenses for magnification was undertaken in 1568 by Damiello Barbaro, while W. Snell (1580-1626), a professor of mathematics at Leiden, in 1624 promulgated the law of refraction. The theory of vision and the concept of the optical decussation was addressed with considerable accuracy by René Descartes (1596-1650) in 1637, while Sir Isaac Newton, A. Haller and Goethe squabbled bitterly about the nature of color. Descartes was of French ancestry, born near Tours and educated initially as a lawyer in Poitiers. He subsequently evolved into a philosopher mathematician and physiologist of exquisite sensitivity and intellectual brilliance. Apart from reconstructing philosophy into a unified system of certain truth modeled on mathematics and supported by rigorous rationalism, he addressed aspects of physiology with novel insight.

The kaleidoscope and lenticular stereoscope were invented by the Scottish physicist, Sir David Brewster (1781-1868) a century later and provided a basis whereby different applications of lenses and color appreciation might be assimilated in a variety of systems such as microscopy, astronomy and chemical science.

The production by Hans Lippershey (1571-1619) of a variety of short and long lenses able to render distant objects near appears to have been a seminal step in the evolution of the science of optics. Thus the design of effective microscopes and telescopes evolved from early simple devices utilized by Leeuwenhoek and Galileo. Subsequent introduction of a compound microscope by Robert Hooke (1635-1703) further expanded the horizon and the production of a reflecting microscope with an improved achromatic objective by G. Amici (1786-1863) in 1812 provided even greater visual acuity. The advent of the 19th century encompassed the disclosure of the binocular microscope (Riddel in 1851), an improved achromatic objective and the oil immersion lens by Ernst Abbe (1840-1905)) in 1878. In daily life the introduction by F. Donders (1818-1889) of modernized spectacles with prismatic and cylindrical lenses and hinged sidepieces considerably altered the perception of members of the public domain. Similarly the construction of complex and sophisticated telescopes amplified the ability of the eye to detect even the outermost planets of the solar system.

"De Homine" (1662), by Descartes (right), is regarded as the first European textbook of physiology and deals with the human body as a material machine directed by a rational soul that Descartes regarded as located in the pineal gland. As an adherent of the Iatromathematical School, that proposed that all physiological phenomena were explicable on the basis of the laws of physics, Descartes was drawn to evaluate the basis of sight. His mathematical acuity enabled him to grasp the optical principles of vision (left) and his anatomic skills defined the significance of the optic chiasma and the decussation of the visual pathways (center bottom).

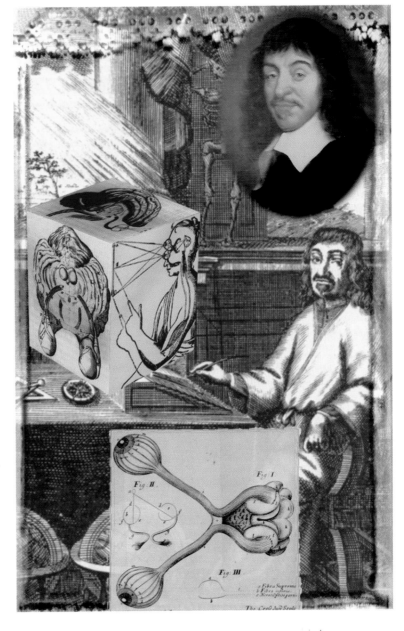

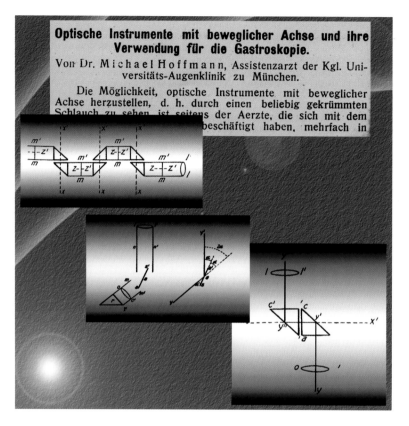

Optische Instrumente mit beweglicher Achse und ihre Verwendung für die Gastroskopie.

Von Dr. Michael Hoffmann, Assistenzarzt der Kgl. Universitäts-Augenklinik zu München.

Die Möglichkeit, optische Instrumente mit beweglicher Achse herzustellen, d. h. durch einen beliebig gekrümmten Schlauch zu sehen, ist seitens der Aerzte, die sich mit dem beschäftigt haben, mehrfach in

Michael Hoffman of Munich was one of the first optical engineers to propose a solution to the problem of bending light around a corner using multiple prisms and lenses (1911). His proposal to apply this concept to gastroscopy (*"Optical Instruments with Moveable Axes and their Application to Gastroscopy"*) (*top*) was originally received with considerable enthusiasm. Unfortunately the delicacy of the design was such that the lenses were easily shifted off their axis during the procedure with consequent loss of visibility.

Although considerable information existed at the end of the 19th century in regard to the science of microscopic and macroscopic technology, considerable difficulties in interfacing lighting and optical systems hampered the development of gastrointestinal endoscopy. In particular the problems inherent in providing adequate illumination and image retention as well as definition were paramount and amplified by the need to incorporate flexibility. Existing endoscopes consisted of a train of copying lenses and intermediate field lenses, which were either rigid or with a limited flexibility. Since the lenses were all of the positive variety, they generated a very large curvature of field and as a result image quality was often poor. The fact that as many as 50 lenses might be used in sequence resulted in poor light transmission and considerable distortion. Light intensity was a critical issue since sources of adequate brilliance were not available and the small aperture needed for acceptable definition further accentuated this problem. Although some of the difficulties appeared surmountable by the introduction of prisms in a moveable tube (*above*) by Michael Hoffman (1911), this design proved impractical since they were easily dislocated during the insertion of the endoscope.

An alternative approach utilized a tube containing a number of very thick lenses with a short focal distance that could be bent to 34 degrees without image distortion and was more serviceable, although still imperfect in terms of image acquisition. Subsequent innovations included altering the angle of view (this eliminated distortion at the image edge and increase the magnification, although at the price of narrowing the image) and the introduction of telescopic optical systems which provided increased magnification (4x) and eliminated problems associated with a lens-tube optical system. Unfortunately the inadequacy of the small bulb light source and multiple lenses resulted in a significant loss of image brilliance and a restricted, narrow field of vision. The combination of this problem and limited flexibility of the device greatly diminished the utility of the endoscope, particularly when employed in a curved organ such as the stomach.

Obvious limitations imposed by standard optical devices were to a large extent the rate-limiting step in the development of endoscopy. Indeed it is fortunate at this juncture that the observations of D. Colladon, J. Babinet and J. Tyndal that light could be conducted down a stream of water were recalled and in 1927, Baird secured a British patent for the idea of transmitting light down a flexible tube. The application of this "well known" concept that that light could be conducted along a curved glass rod due to multiple total internal reflections at the walls of this instrument was however never pursued in its entirety. It would in fact require a further three decades before the idea of "fiber-optics" was further explored by H. Hopkins and N. S. Kapany.

N. S. Kapany, while a graduate student at Imperial College, London, was able to derive a theory as well as to demonstrate in practice what had previously thought to be impossible. Namely that a fiber of less than 10-12 wavelengths (approx. 1 micron) in diameter could be used to successfully transmit light. The second step was provided in 1954, when H. Hopkins, a professor in Applied Optics at the University of Reading, England, who had focused on the mathematical processes of optical design, devised an optical unit which could convey optical images along a flexible axis.

Unfortunately for Hopkins, neither corporate nor scientific support for his design could be identified in either England or the United States. Indeed considerable reservations were expressed as to the utility of the early rod-lens system that he proposed, since it was inferior to the conventional lens system of the day in terms of optical quality given the poor picture quality produced by glass fibers. Fortunately Karl Storz (1911-1996) suggested to Hopkins the concept of fiber-optic light transmission coupled with a rod-lens optical system. This system used glass rods instead of small lenses within the optical shaft, and thereby allowed for improved resolution, contrast and brightness as well as a wide-field viewing angle while maintaining an appropriately small diameter. Illumination was supplied by a bright light source, separate from the viewing instrument, with light transmission through glass fibers along the shaft of the instrument.

Based upon an appreciation of the possible application of the optical principles enunciated by the work of Hopkins and Kapany, Basil Hirschowitz had expanded upon the concept and produced a flexible fiberglass endoscope that incorporated a parallel array of organized glass fibers with a light bulb at the distal end. Although objects could be visualized with this system, initial problems with the fiber bundles alignment and coating resulted in a transmitted grainy image unsuitable for

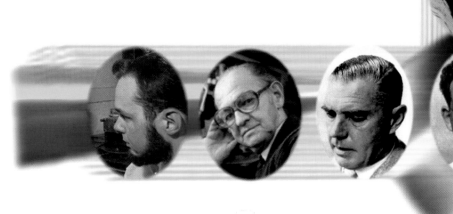

The Men who bent the Light (from top to bottom left). Daniel Colladon of Geneva (1841) was the first to demonstrate light guiding using jets of cascading water. Jacques Babinet adapted this technique and demonstrated that it could be undertaken in glass rods but by his death in 1872 had not pursued the issue even though he had suggested that such a device might be used to "light up the mouth". At the suggestion of M. Faraday, J. Tyndall performed experiments (1853) in London to show the phenomenon of light bending, but omitted to indicate his lack of primacy in the area. While a medical student in Munich (1930) H. Lamm successfully transmitted images through glass fibers. Abraham van Heel, a Dutch physicist, produced the first bundles of clad fibers for image transmission (1952) although a year previously Holger Møller Hansen of Denmark had applied for a Danish patent on a "flexible picture transport cable." Larry Curtiss of the University of Ann Arbor, Michigan, made the first glass clad fibers to be used in Hirschowitz gastroscope.

H. Hopkins (*right*), a professor of Applied Optics at Imperial College and subsequently the University of Reading, England was a gifted scientist who apart from his contributions to the establishment of fiber optic systems was responsible for the development of the diffraction theory of image formation. Although initially recognized for his invention of the zoom lens (1945) his work on the rod-lens optical system which he patented (Great Britain #954629) in 1959 is now recognized as of fundamental importance. N. S. Kapany (*left*), while a graduate student at Imperial College, London, was able to demonstrate that a glass fiber of one micron could successfully convey light. Together with Hopkins, an optical unit was designed (*right*) which could convey images along a flexible axis.

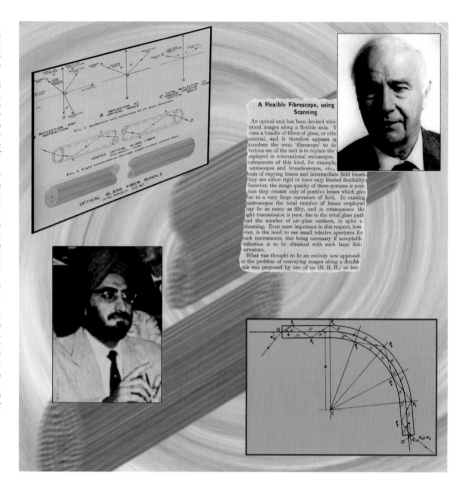

clinical usage. A variety of difficulties including fiber quality and orientation were resolved by Curtiss and Hirschowitz, enabling the development of a viable fiber-optic endoscope and introducing a new era of vision which successfully encompassed both the issues of flexibility and adequate image acquisition. Subsequent development of dynamic scanning and spatial filtering improved resolution significantly and the further elaboration of charge coupled devices once again amplified the quality of the imagery as electronic and computer assisted technology propelled by flexibility advanced beyond the previous boundaries established by anatomical and technical limitations. The evolution of optics coupled to the 20th century marriage of two different forms of glass, simple lenses and a bundle of fibers, generated an endoscope capable of enlightening the insides of even the most curious of men.

The Metamorphosis–Rigid to Flexible (1900–1930) | CHAPTER 4

INTRODUCTION

By the turn of the century, with electricity in place, adequate lighting, good concepts of sedation and lenses and engineering had evolved to the point that a serious approach to appropriate and adequate visualization could be undertaken.

In general the development of endoscopic instrumentation between 1900 and 1930 evolved within the constraints of three different categories each loosely governed by overlapping principles: (1) Open tube systems, (2) Rigid tubes with added optical systems, and (3) Flexible tubes that could be straightened after introduction into the stomach. Instruments of this period exhibited heterogeneity of construction and a melange of design often incompatible with their stated purpose. The cause of this conceptual obfuscation reflected in many instances the limited series of clinical studies available for review of efficacy and the fact that much work appeared to be based more upon theoretical considerations and clinical empiricism rather than rigorous and systematic study.

OPEN TUBE INSTRUMENTS

After the initial contributions of Kussmaul, the development of gastroscopy became closely associated with esophagoscopy. Chevalier Jackson (1907) of Philadelphia and W. Hill and Herschel (1911) of England were among the early esophagoscopists, who proposed that the stomach could be quite adequately and safely examined utilizing open tubes. For the most part their proposals met with little general acceptance, since it was evident that special skill was necessary to obtain the superlative results that they presented.

Jackson, despite being an otorhinolaryngologist, became adept at inspection of the stomach through an open tube devoid of any optical system and differing only from an esophagoscope in its increased length. Narcosis was employed and the patient maintained in a recumbent position throughout the procedure. Although there was no apparatus for inflation of the stomach, visibility was good since residual gastric fluid could be removed by continuous suction through a narrow tube attached to the outer surface of the instrument. Jackson claimed that each examination lasted about 30 minutes and within that time he could in most

It is unlikely that Hippocrates as he sat under the sun-dappled tree in Kos could have conceived of diagnosis moving beyond the palpating hand to the illumination of the interior.

To provide light, specula and sunlit mirrors yielded to tubes, candles, lamps and finally carbon and platinum electric filaments. For vision, single lenses became multiple and were augmented with prisms and finally supplanted by fibers. To turn the corner physicians sought flexibility and discarded rigid instruments to facilitate ingress to the furthermost recesses of the stomach. This metamorphosis of diagnosis from the digit to the macula involved not only physicians but also optical, electrical and structural engineers as well as corporations and in many instances, courage.

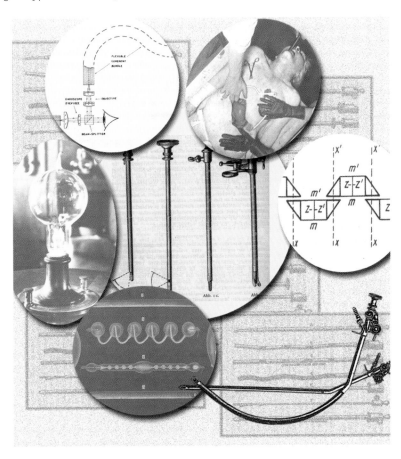

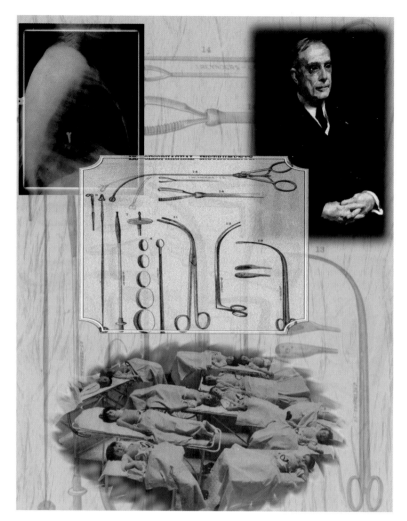

Chevalier Jackson of Philadelphia (*top right*), apart from his talents as a sculptor, writer and painter, was an esophagoscopist of virtuoso-like skill. Able to maneuver the rigid esophagoscope with the dexterity of a maestro he developed a wide range of instruments (*center*) for the extraction of foreign bodies (*top left*). Innumerable children (patients from his ward bottom) were saved by his therapeutic endeavors and to this day the manufacture of the size/shape configurations of toys in the USA is measured against the huge collection he removed over his career. Given his consummate skill with the rigid endoscope he asserted that it was adequate for gastroscopy and initially criticized the efforts to introduce bent or flexible devices.

patients examine 50-75% of the mucosa. In his first series he reported visualization of the pylorus in 2 of 17 individuals and when the stomach was maneuvered by palpation through the external abdominal wall he was able to even biopsy a pyloric tumor. Published roentgenograms of the procedure dramatically demonstrated the considerable mobility of the tip of the instrument. Although Jackson was a man of considerable conviction and consummate endoscopic skill, as attested to by his vast experience at foreign body removal and biopsy proven diagnosis, the limitations of view afforded by his technique mitigated against its general acceptance.

In England the gastroenterologist Herschel, working in conjunction with the otolaryngeal surgeon, W. Hill, described their success with a slightly modified technique. Concerned at the use of a "blind introduction" they utilized an open tube inserted into the stomach under direct visual control. In addition to facilitate visualization of the stomach they utilized both insufflation and an optical system with a lamp.

Although Jackson and Hill emphasized the importance of visual control while introducing the instrument, and were acknowledged to possess considerable dexterity in this maneuver, most contemporary gastroscopists introduced their open-tube instruments blindly unless resistance was encountered. Thus a wide variety of obturators, elastic bougies or long flexible rubber tips were generally employed to facilitate introduction of the gastroscope. Despite the enthusiasm of Hill and Jackson, subsequent development of endoscopes over the next two decades followed the principle of a rigid tube through which an optical system was passed.

RIGID TUBES WITH OPTICAL SYSTEMS

Although the instrument designed by Rosenheim was not generally accepted, his demonstration that straight instruments could be effectively utilized to view the stomach was recognized as an important contribution. Perforations that were associated however mandated the development of a safer mode of instrument introduction. As a result in the period following his publications straight optical systems were passed through soft outer tubes introduced in the stomach in order to avoid perforation of the lower part of the esophagus. Of note was the fact that such instruments were introduced blindly and only after 1911 were a variety of straight rigid gastroscopes used again.

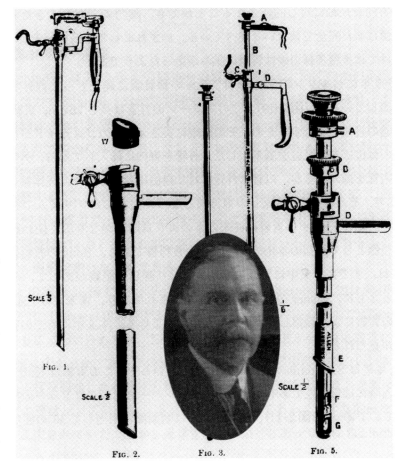

A diverse group of such instruments was described and details of some are worthy of note. In 1908 K. Loening (1877-1926) and Stieda of Halle designed a gastroscope that consisted of an outer soft rubber tube that was introduced in the stomach with the aid of an obturator. Once placement was considered adequate, a straight optical system carrying the lamp was inserted via the outer tube. This device was considered reasonably safe and although some perforations were reported early in its development it was used by others.

Heynemann of Berlin paid particular attention to the optical system and his instrument was also judged to be of high quality. In fact the Hill instrument utilized the optical system designed by Heynemann.

W. Kausch (1867-1928) in 1909 reported the details of a gastroscope that he had designed which possessed an outer elastic tube into which a straight optical system was placed. He subsequently in 1922 included an ingenious idea of inserting a prism window to regulate the optics for anterior and posterior viewing, but this proved impractical and did not attain commercial acceptance. Although Collens and Gray revisited the principle of a flexible outer tube and a straight optical system in 1928, minimal progress was made and the concept languished. A gastroscope produced in London by Souttar and Thompson in 1909 at the same time as that of Kausch comprised a rigid tube that possessed an angle at the pharynx and one at the cardia. As a result of criticism by Hill it was modified and the pharyngeal angle removed. Nevertheless it proved unsafe and a number of fatal perforations were reported.

Dissatisfied with the current instrumentation available for access to the stomach, a number of physicians including Kelling, T. Rovsing (1862-1927), Lindstedt, Thinius and C. Beck (1864-1916) utilized cystoscopes and even laparoscopes to obtain better results. Such endeavors however met with little success and this line of thought was not pursued.

FLEXIBLE TUBES STRAIGHTENED AFTER INTRODUCTION

Kelling of Dresden (1898) was the chief proponent of the concept of flexible tubes that could be straightened after introduction into the stomach, while Kuttner (1897) and Sussmann (1911) in Berlin provided further sup-

The Loening—Stieda endoscope (1908). This device sought to obviate the danger of perforation by preliminary introduction of a flexible soft outer tube and obturator (left) followed by the subsequent insertion of the optical system.

The English otolaryngeal surgeon, W. Hill (bottom), in conjunction with Herschel (a gastroenterologist), devised a complex and highly effective endoscope (1908) (background) that could be used both for esophageal and gastric procedures. To facilitate gastric visualization they added an insufflation channel in addition to the lamp and magnification lenses.

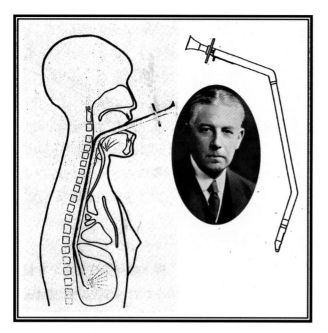

H. J. Souttar (*center*) modified the endoscope with a series of angles to facilitate introduction. Although potentially useful, the rigidity of the angulation proved ungainly and a number of perforations followed by serious criticism led to its withdrawal from usage.

port for this proposal. Although it was innovative and a forerunner in the field, the gastroscope designed by Kuttner was regarded as impractical and not used by others. The device was slightly flexible in its entire length and contained a built-in optic, but problems with straightening and poor visibility doomed its success. Indeed the overall difficulties encountered with this class of contrivance were posed by the fact that in many instances straightening was either impossible, incomplete or could be only achieved by force. As a result none of these instruments was deemed adequate for clinical use, and the idea was not pursued.

The gastroscope designed by Sussmann, although a technical masterpiece, was expensive and although easy to introduce was fragile and often needed repair. The device possessed a slight angle in its rigid part at the level of the pharynx and was flexible only in the distal part that contained a glass tip. Of particular utility was the fact that the window of the optical system could be rotated for inspection in various directions. However, the picture was often blurred because of a slight dislocation of the lenses. A further problem encountered was that when the optical system window became soiled the entire instrument had to be removed for cleaning. Although the instrument often straightened itself after introduction occasionally there was difficulty and the straightening maneuver caused pain. The examination was undertaken with the patient in right lateral position (radiographs had demonstrated the instrument to be the least flexed in this position) and the stomach was inflated with compressed air or oxygen from a cylinder.

THE INTRODUCTION OF FLEXIBILITY: 1911-1932

Despite the creativity of engineers and the resourcefulness of physicians the two decades after 1911 were dominated by the principle of straight rigid tubes with optical systems until 1932, when Schindler introduced the flexible gastroscope. During this period the two instruments of most efficacy were the gastroscopes of Elsner in Berlin (1911) and Schindler (1922) in Munich.

The gastroscope produced by Elsner was reported as safe and effective such that in 1921 a series of 500 examinations using the Elsner gastroscope without any complication were described. In addition it produced an image that was so bright and sharp that the first successful gastroscopic pictures were taken through it. It thus remained the dominant instrument until Schindler introduced his own design some ten years later. The Elsner gastroscope was to a certain extent modeled on a cystoscope and was straight with a rubber tip and an optical system that could be introduced through the outer tube that carried the lamp at the tip. Although the window of the optical system could be protected by turning the inner tube, it was relatively easily soiled, and represented one of the major disadvantages of the instrument. As a result, in 1923, Elsner produced an improved model in which he added an air tube that could be used to clean the optical window.

The Schindler Gastroscope

The rigid gastroscope introduced by R. Schindler in 1922 and although slightly modified by others, was the most extensively used instrument of the decade up to 1932, when the "flexible" gastroscope first became a reality. Indeed most of the fundamental observations of gastroscopy were undertaken with this device and its contributions to the resolution of various diseases of the stomach probably make this instrument one of the great bio-technical devices of the century. The rigid gastroscope as first designed by Schindler in 1922 consisted of a straight open outer tube introduced into the stomach with an obturator on whose tip a long (8 cm) rubber finger had been implanted to ensure safe guidance during introduction. Once the

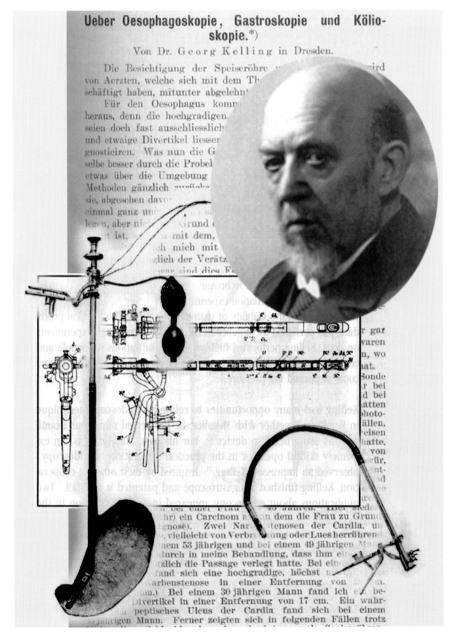

George Kelling (*top right*) of Dresden, although better remembered for his contributions to the establishment of laparoscopy, played a role in the evolution of gastroscopy. The Kelling gastroscope (*center*) was a masterpiece of engineering craft, but its utility was limited due to its complexity. The outer tube carried a lamp and the distal part of the tube possessed a segmental flexibility and could be straightened by a complicated mechanism when introduced in the stomach, after which a straight optical system was inserted via the outer tube. The tip of the instrument was slightly angled (*bottom left*), since this was thought to facilitate a more detailed inspection of the antrum than a straight instrument. Although Kelling examined more than thirty patients and published his observations, the device was poorly received by his colleagues and no other physician adopted its usage.

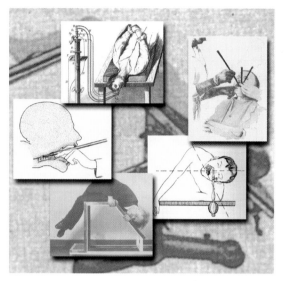

Examination Modes. There was considerable debate regarding the best clinical application of the instruments. Each expert proposed examination in variety of positions that ranged from sitting, to horizontal either supine or prone in the right or even left lateral position. Even the knee-chest position had its proponents! Some authors introduced their instrument with the patient sitting, but then continued the examination in horizontal position to obviate problems encountered with regurgitation. Although general anesthesia was occasionally used, morphine, scopolamine and other sedatives were most commonly utilized. Local anesthesia of the pharynx with cocaine was a later introduction that proved of considerable use in facilitating instrumentation. Almost all gastroscopists inflated the stomach with air, carbon dioxide or oxygen except for C. Jackson, who examined without any inflation. Although water filling had been evaluated, poor visibility and aspiration had led to disenchantment with this technique.

stomach had been safely reached the optical tube that carried the lamp was then utilized to replace the obturator.

Experience was a critical determinant in usage and Schindler's initial reports document successful gastric introduction in 97% of patients, but examination was only possible in 55% with pyloric visibility in 20% and two fatal perforations occurred. Others such as Gutzeit reported in his first five hundred cases a successful introduction rate that varied from 80-95 % and adequate examination in two thirds of the patients with no accidents. Indeed many reports of the time indicate that perforations with the Schindler instrument were rare and its design was generally recognized as superior. The subsequent renown of Schindler was based principally upon his *"Lehrbuch und Atlas der Gastroskopie"* of 1923, that was unique both in its pictures and descriptions of a wide variety of stomach conditions. For the first time gastroenterologists could see what they were treating and even monitor the effects of their therapy. The visual recognition of gastric pathology thus became an important facet of gastroenterology and necessary for the successful diagnosis and management of disease.

In 1923, shortly after the introduction of the Schindler gastroscope, W. Sternberg also of Munich introduced a similar instrument that he vociferously claimed to be of greater efficacy. The device was of a smaller diameter, resembled a cystoscope, and was introduced with the patient in the unusual knee-elbow position. Although Sternberg claimed to have undertaken an enormous number of examinations with minimal morbidity, Schindler resoundingly condemned his instrument and technique. In this judgement he was subsequently proved correct when Sternberg in 1923 mortally injured a patient at a demonstration to E. Ferdinand Sauerbruch (1875-1951) in Munich at a meeting of the Bavarian Surgical Association. Sauerbruch had invited both Schindler and Sternberg to his clinic to demonstrate their instruments and techniques at the meeting in the presence of a number of surgeons. Schindler declined to appear lest he be associated with Sternberg whose metal tipped instrument he considered unsafe. Although the patient was unsuitable for the purpose of the demonstration, Sternberg persisted despite considerable difficulty in introducing the instrument, which finally could not be accomplished. Twelve hours later the patient had developed symptoms of a serious mediastinitis and despite cervical exploration perished from what was referred to as a "retro-esophageal phlegmon" consequent upon a partial rupture of the upper esophagus.

Sauerbruch lost no time in publishing the case, using the fatal outcome as strong argument against gastroscopy. As a consequence of this attack on gastroscopy by a surgeon of Sauerbruch's influence, the discipline of gastroscopy suffered a severe setback as surgeons now opposed the technique and challenged its safety. Nevertheless when Gottstein reviewed the published reports of 2,500 gastroscopy results in 1926 only 15 fatal perforations were noted. Additional information available in the same year from a questionnaire by Hubner to sixteen well-known gastroscopists revealed that in a total of 3,627 examinations there had been nine accidents and a mortality of 0.2-0.3 %. The spread of expertise combined with the increased experience overall resulted in considerable decline in accidents and despite opposition the procedure enjoyed a generally good reputation.

In 1922 the five types of gastroscope available included those constructed by Sussman, Loening-Stieda, Elsner, Schindler and Kausch. Thereafter Gottstein (1924), Hubner (1926) and Korbsch had variously produced instruments that were permutations of previous models. Of these the Korbsch instrument (Berlin,

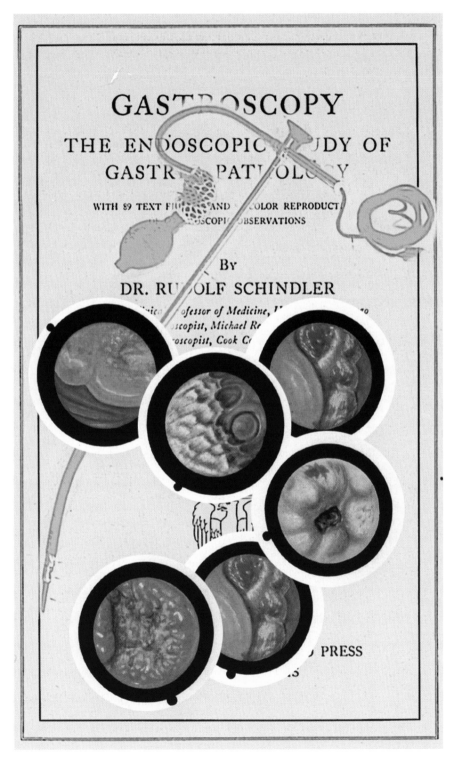

The English translation (1937) of R. Schindler's seminal text *"Lehrbuch und Atlas der Gastroskopie"*. Rudolf Schindler of Munich had during his military service become intrigued with the prevalence of the vague diagnosis of gastritis amongst the soldiers. Frustrated by his inability to adequately visualize the stomach he devised a rigid gastroscope (1922) and published his findings *"Problems and Techniques of Gastroscopy with a description of a new Gastroscope"* (Arch. VerdauKr., 1922, 30, 133-66.). A year later (1923) he published a book, *"Lehrbuch und Atlas der Gastroskopie"*, that was unique in its color pictures (*center*) and descriptions of gastric pathology. Schindler personally supervised the hand painted illustrations and the cost of the color plates for the text was underwritten by the generosity of a former patient, Mrs. Morse of Chicago. After his forced to the United States in 1934 this text was translated with the aid of Walter L Palmer of the University of Chicago and in 1937 published as *"Gastroscopy, The Endoscopic Study of Gastric Pathology"*.

Some examples of the diversity of gastroscopes available between 1911-1933. The Elsner scope (1911) (top) was the most widely used prior to the introduction of the Schindler rigid gastroscope (2nd) in 1922. The Sternberg instrument (3rd) introduced in 1923 was claimed to have a size advantage (9mm as compared to 11mm of the preceding two) as well as better visibility. The Korbsch instrument of 1926 (4th) had an even smaller diameter of 8-5 mm but was supplanted in 1932 by the Schindler flexible instrument (5th). The disadvantage of its relatively large diameter (12 mm) was far outweighed by the unique introduction of flexibility. Korbsch subsequently produced a smaller elastic metal instrument (1933) (bottom) but the Schindler design became the accepted gastroscope of the decade.

1925) had enjoyed brief popularity as a slimmer (7mm) version of the Elsner instrument with the addition of a slightly angled tip. Thus, by 1931, although there were no less than seven types of gastroscope available (Elsner, Sternberg, Schindler, modified Hohlweg-Schindler, Korbsch, Hubner and Bensaude), none was risk free. Indeed all were cumbersome to use and considerable expertise was required not only to ensure safety but also to gain adequate information. It was therefore apparent to all and especially Schindler that such issues could only be resolved if a flexible instrument with appropriately modified optics could be developed. Thus between 1928 and 1932 Schindler in conjunction with Georg Wolf, the skilled instrument manufacturer of Berlin, sought to overcome the problems of visibility and maneuverability posed by rigidity.

Both Wolf and Schindler agreed that the Sussman instrument constructed by Wolf was flawed since "the conceptions upon which its construction was based were wrong!" Schindler was quick to point out that "...the straightening procedure was very dangerous and the optical system was easily dislocated." Their collaboration began in 1928 and despite an initial design of a fully flexible gastroscope moved at Schindler's insistence towards a semi-flexible instrument. This decision was based upon the earlier work of Hoffmann in Munich, who had seventeen years previously proposed the incorporation of prisms in a movable tube to resolve the optical problems of rigidity. Based upon Hoffmann's earlier work, Schindler determined that the proposed endoscope would need to be flexible from a point 3cm above the cardia.

THE SEMI-FLEXIBLE ENDOSCOPE

The first attempt to construct a flexible gastroscope was undertaken by Hoffmann in 1911 based upon the recognition that an optical image could be conducted by a number of movable prisms that enabled the instrument to be flexed. Wolf, after his disappointing experience with the Sussman gastroscope, had attempted to utilize this movable tube and prism design but to no avail. Unfortunately the optical principles of this instrument were not adequate for clinical use and only data obtained in cadaver studies were published. However in 1919, Lange at the

Berlin factory of Goertz discovered and patented his observation that it was possible to visualize objects through a curved tube containing a number of lenses of short focal length. In so doing he resolved the principle issue of how an image might be transmitted around the bend created by a flexed instrument. This discovery allowed an optical image produced by a lens of short focal distance to be repeatedly reproduced by a number of collecting lenses of great refractive power and thereby conveyed to the level of the ocular lens for inspection by the viewer.

Schindler, who had by 1932 had acquired more than a decade of experience in both instrument use and design, was not slow in perceiving what was required. Similarly Wolf, a Berlin instrument maker, had already constructed the rigid endoscopes of Elsner, Sternberg, Sussmann and Hohlweg and was possessed of considerable familiarity with the field. Working in conjunction, Schindler and Wolf constructed (after six versions) and patented by 1932 a flexible gastroscope. Within a short time its efficacy and safety had become common knowledge.

Although the first version of the new gastroscope was flexible in its entire length, it proved more satisfactory to have only the distal half flexible with the ocular half maintained rigid and straight. This facilitated introduction of the instrument into the stomach, and also enabled simplification of the design of the optical system. In addition the flexible part was made elastic and could straighten itself and the rubber fingertip was retained and modified from the original rigid instrument to facilitate safe passage. Thus the final model of the instrument consisted of a straight rigid proximal part and a distal flexible segment that contained a number of lenses of short focal length capable of transmitting the optical image even when the instrument was flexed. Even when bent in a number of different planes an undistorted image could be obtained provided the angle did not exceed 34°. The window of the optical system was constructed flat and elevated, to enable the window to be cleaned by rotating the instrument against the stomach wall. Although this was satisfactory it was inferior to the rigid gastroscope where the optical system could be removed for cleaning. The addition of a sponge rubber tip to wipe off the esophageal mucus and prevent the optic from being soiled was proposed but proved to be unsafe and caused gastric perforations. A rubber ball tip, like the original fingertip, therefore replaced it, and was safe. Although the flexible optical system was somewhat inferior to the excellent systems of some of the rigid instruments, the current design of the gastroscope rendered it not only easy to pass into the stomach, but also safe. As a result of these dramatic advances the use of the gastroscope became widely accepted in many countries, and culminated in a rapid, almost explosive, spread of the "gastroscopic method" that had for so long languished in the netherworld of unfulfilled discoveries.

The introduction of the flexible gastroscope for the most part eliminated the risk of perforation of the lower part of the esophagus, where rigid instruments had caused damage. The technique of examination, developed with the rigid instrument, was easily adapted for the flexible gastroscope and the distal part of the stomach could be inspected in about 80 % of patients.

The Sussman gastroscope designed by Wolf of Berlin (1912). Based upon the original proposal of Hoffman in 1911 that moveable prisms and lenses could be used to manufacture a flexible gastroscope, the instrument maker, Georg Wolf, had in collaboration with Sussman designed an endoscope capable of flexion. A complex system of pulleys, screws and levers were incorporated to facilitate this, but the concept was marred by the overly exquisite delicacy of design and the ease with which the lenses became displaced.

Apart from the danger of perforation associated with the use of the rigid gastroscope, a critical problem was posed by the lack of adequate visibility of large areas of the stomach. Thus substantial zones (1-4) in the cardia, body and antrum were invisible to the endoscopist.

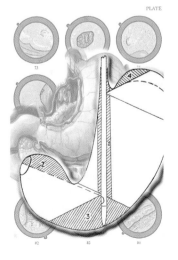

PLATE

The Schindler-Wolf semi-flexible gastroscope c. 1932. The relationship between Schindler and Wolf reflected the belief of both parties in the need for a flexible gastroscope. The design parameters sought were a thin flexible tube whose length and flexibility would not only enable lenses to be mounted in such a fashion that flexion would not interfere with vision but provide adequate length to examine the stomach. Ultimately, in order to accommodate these criteria and satisfy the perfection that Schindler sought, Wolf was forced to produce six gastroscope prototypes between 1928 and 1932! On July 13, 1930 patent #629,590 was awarded to Georg Wolf for the development of the first fully flexible gastroscope, which contained a sequence of lenses screwed to the sides of the tube. A further modification resulted in yet another patent filing and on July 7th, 1932 patent #662,788 was similarly awarded to Wolf for his design of the semi-flexible gastroscope. The latter model was unique in that it contained lenses, which were displaceable along the interior of the tube following the transmission of an elastic pressure provided by a bronze coil located at the distal end. Thus increasing the tension on the coil allowed the lenses to be pushed against the upper end into a space separating the rigid and flexible segments. Such was the success of this design that the introduction of the instrument resulted in "...a rapid, almost explosive, spread of the gastroscopic method". Not unaware of the staggering potential of his device, Wolf had within three years successfully applied for and received a U.S. patent for this gastroscope and on March 17, 1935 the semi-flexible gastroscope was awarded U.S. patent #1,995,196.

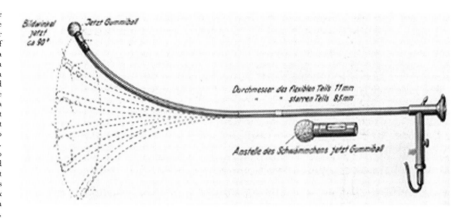

HEINRICH LAMM

It is interesting to note that the Schindler semi-flexible gastroscope saga might have been very much different. Heinrich Lamm, while a medical student at Munich, had the opportunity to observe Schindler demonstrate his gastroscope and concluded that it lacked adequate flexibility. Possessed of a keen intelligence he concluded that the logical solution would be the use of flexible glass fibers. Although he knew little about internal reflection, he surmised that thin rods of quartz or a bundle of glass fibers could carry an image point by point if the fibers were coherently arranged. Believing that a real image could be transmitted "point by point" from one surface of a fiber to another he proposed that a bundle of fibers would convey an image accurately if the terminal surface was aligned and viewed through an ocular lens. Although only a third-year medical student, Lamm persuaded Schindler to fund the project and subsequently obtained help from Walter Gerlach, a prominent physicist who subsequently became involved in the German atomic bomb program. Lamm purchased glass fibers from the G. Rodenstock Optical Works (this translates serendipitously as "clear stick"). Having combed the glass threads into a bundle he successfully demonstrated that light could follow a curved path. To confirm his results he focused the bright light from a V shaped filament of a frosted bulb onto one end of the bundle and demonstrated a faint V image of the filament at the other end. This picture was recorded on photographic film and although the glass was not clear and the fibers imperfectly aligned remains the first example of a fiber optic transmitted image. Elated at the possibilities of his work, Lamm filed a patent with the German patent office only to find that one had already been granted to Clarence Hansell (US Patent 1,751,584-Picture Transmission). The Marconi Company who owned the British license informed him that neither they nor Hansell had "tried to utilize the principle." Undeterred, Lamm published his work as sole author under the title of "*Biegsame optische Geräte*" (Flexible Fiber Optic Instruments) in the October 1930 issue of the *Zeitschrift für Instrumentenkunde*. The unusual event of lone authorship in Germany of this time period may be interpreted as evidence of Schindler's lack of confidence in the work or his consideration that the experiments had failed. In his paper Lamm however stated "the experimental proof of the possibility to transmit images through a flexible multi-fiber a conductor of radiant energy justifies this communication". He presciently concluded "I also hope that some optical firm possessed of more means, sources of supply and experience than I have could be induced by this report to build a serviceable flexible gastroscope."

Unfortunately Lamm was Jewish and the rise of Adolf Hitler precluded his further medical and scientific progress in Europe. Having completed his residency at the Jewish hospital in Breslau he and his physician wife fled Germany reaching America in 1937, where he obtained a position in a psychiatry hospital in Kansas City. Desperate to pursue his vocation as a surgeon he finally found residence in a town of 1,500 person at the southern tip of Texas and his great mind that might have altered the face of endoscopy languished far from the pinnacles of power and intellect. Schindler, though aware of Lamm's presence in the USA, did not pursue further contact with him. Indeed when presented with the details of the first fiber-optic gastroscope some thirty years later, he recalled that Lamm had proposed the idea in 1928-9 but that "they" (Lamm and he) had failed due to lack of adequate coating of the glass bundles and the modest input of physicists!

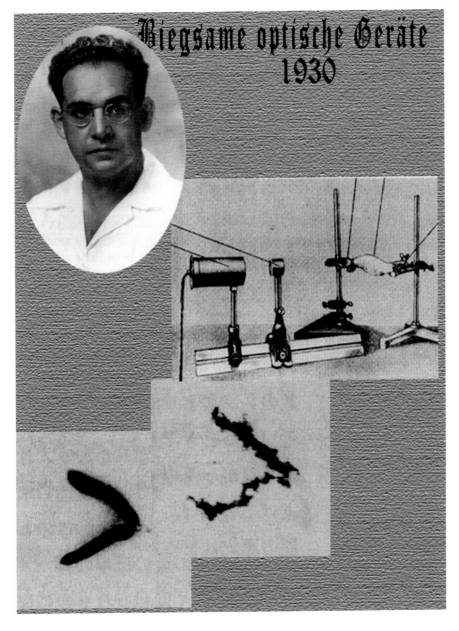

Biegsame optische Geräte 1930

The apparatus (*right*) used by Heinrich Lamm (*left*) in 1930, as a 22-year medical student in Munich, to prove that a bundle of glass fibers could transmit the image of a light bulb filament around a bend. The V shaped bare filament image (*bottom left*) was transmitted through a crudely constructed bundle of glass fibers and generated a spotty but recognizable image (*right*) which he recorded on photographic film for posterity.

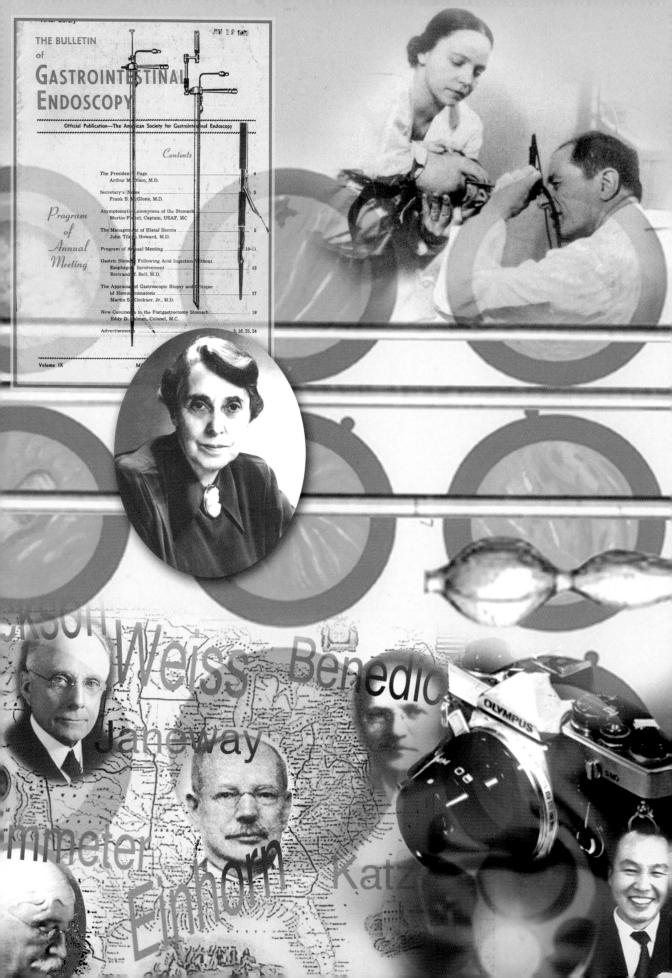

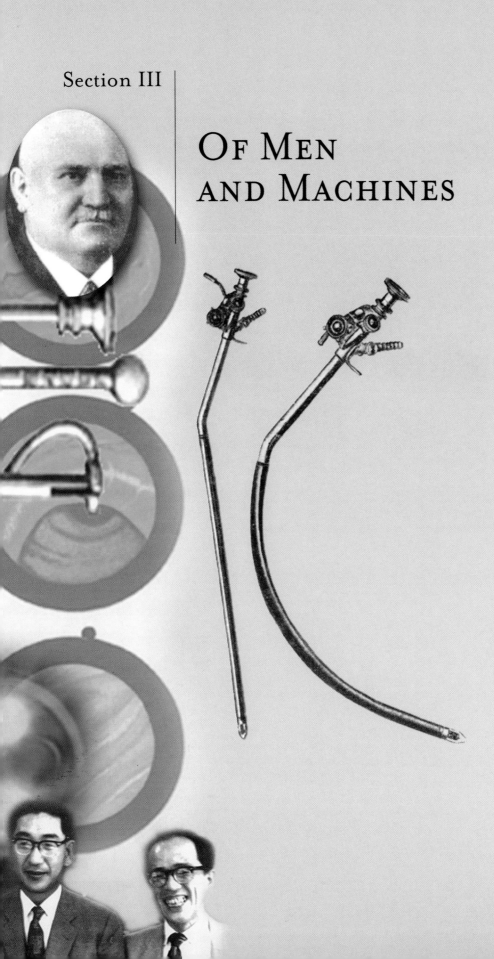

OF MEN
AND MACHINES

| *Rudolf Schindler*

68

A̶LTHOUGH   THE   DEVELOPMENT   of
gastroscopy owed a great debt to numerous individuals, there is little doubt that credit for its dramatic evolution in the 20th century reflects the role of Rudolf Schindler.

While sporadic success had marked the contributions of Adolph Kussmaul
(1868), Max Nitze, Joseph Leiter (1876) and Johann von Mikulicz-Radecki (1881), it
was Schindler who provided a sustained and consistent advance in both the technology and practice of gastroscopy. The early pioneers of Austro-German endoscopy had

As a result of having
been incarcerated in
Dachau, Schindler and
his family immigrated to
Chicago in the summer
of 1934. A special visa
and appointment to the
faculty of the University
of Chicago was arranged
by Dr. Ortmayer, who
had become a close
friend of Schindler in
Vienna, and Walter
Palmer, the Chief of the
Department of
Gastroenterology.
George Baehr,
Chairman of the
Refugee Physician's
Fund, Mrs. Morse (a
former patient) and
Mrs. Martha Fischer of
Chicago provided
support for the
relocation of the family.

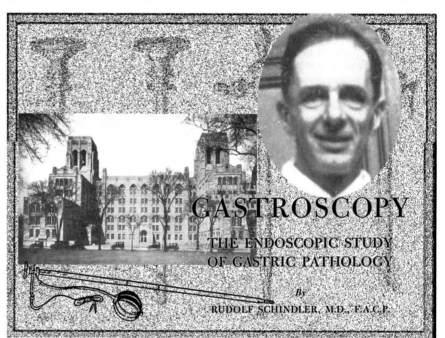

been stimulated not only by the development of the cystoscope and the dexterity of
sword swallowers, but by the obvious need to penetrate the diagnostic darkness of the
luminal void posed by the gastrointestinal tract. Unfortunately the first rigid hollow
tubes lighted by an external headlight provided poor visibility and were dangerous to
insert. The subsequent developments of a light carrier and an illuminating lamp that
could be passed through the tube into the stomach were more useful, but the absence
of lenses resulted in the generation of only a limited view of the gastric lumen. Such
tubes, although serviceable in the extraction of foreign bodies were of marginal usage
in the identification of mucosal detail and anything less than overt pathology. In this
respect endoscopy of the stomach posed a particular problem since the asymmetrical
shape of the cavity required both an objective lens of variable focus and considerable
illumination. Mindful of these parameters, Leiter, the Viennese instrument maker
who had initially been involved in the production of a cystoscope with Nitze, had proposed that the development of a similar optical gastroscope would be necessary to ful-
fil such criteria. The drawback of this instrument was the fact that the optical tube was
unable to be flexed, since lens technology of the time was limited. As a result bending
of the instrument resulted in initial distortion and thereafter with further flexion,

actual obliteration of the image. A further drawback of such rigid instrumentation was not only the difficulty of insertion, but also the likelihood of perforation. Thus, despite a series of thoughtful modifications of the instrument design as well as careful assessment of esophago-gastric anatomy in both cadavers and human patients, the procedure remained both limited and dangerous in its application until the advent of Schindler.

EARLY DAYS

Rudolf Schindler was born in Berlin on May the 10th, 1888, the son of a Jewish banker (Richard) and an artistically gifted Lutheran mother (Martha Simon). Raised in a cultured and sophisticated background, his early interests included poetry, natural history and classical music. Having studied at the Kaiser Wilhelm Gymnasium in Berlin, he graduated in 1905 and thereafter moved to the University of Freiburg. Influenced by his uncle, Richard Simon, who was a Berlin ophthalmologist, Schindler studied medicine, although natural history and marine zoology were of particular interest to him. During his medical training Schindler received, as was the European custom, a broad general medical education and in addition became particularly adept in the area of histology. The latter skill would serve as a basis for his subsequent interest in the elucidation of gastric physiology and pathology, especially gastritis.

After graduating from medical school, the young Schindler became battalion surgeon and pathologist of the 12th Bavarian Infantry Regiment in the 6th Army of the World War I German armed forces. It was during this period that his interest in the gastrointestinal tract was aroused. His curiosity was piqued by the pervasive inability to identify any cause for the common abdominal complaints that soldiers suffered from, as well as the question of whether there existed an organic or even gastric basis for such problems. Schindler concluded that many of the gastrointestinal maladies of the soldiers were diet related and indeed following his own bout with dysentery, he became further convinced of the relationship between military service and gastric disease. This almost obsessional preoccupation with gastric disease, gastritis and military personnel would remain a consistent feature of his future clinical focus. Indeed in the subsequent years he would utilize the gastroscope to demonstrate that military service both initiated and exacerbated certain types of gastric disease.

At the termination of the war, Schindler accepted an appointment in the Schwabing Hospital at Munich and by 1920 had become expert in the use of the rigid Elsner gastroscope. Dissatisfied with the technical characteristics of this instrument, Schindler arranged for the manufacture of his own endoscope by the firm of Reinger, Gebbert and Schall in Munich. With this instrument he assiduously investigated the vast morass of vague and undiagnosed stomach disease that he believed was caused by different types of gastritis.

In 1922 at the age of 34, Schindler married Gabriele Winkler, who although untrained in the medical profession

A street view of Munich c. 1920. During his medical military service in the 12th Bavarian Infantry Regiment of the German Army (1914-1918), Schindler had become particularly interested in the severe and inexplicable gastric problems prevalent amongst the soldiers. It is interesting to note that an Austrian corporal (16th Bavarian Reserve Infantry) of the army at this time, Alois Schiklgruber, aka Adolf Hitler (*the soldier on the right, bottom left*) subsequently documented his symptomatology and its accentuation by incarceration in a classic text on political dyspepsia (*Mein Kampf*). It is likely that *H.Pylori* (*top right*) as well as the stress of trench warfare were implicated in the genesis of "military gastritis". Schindler proposed that such "gastric disorders" could only be adequately investigated if the pathology could be defined and from this conviction sprang his interest in the development of a safe and usable gastroscope. Ironically two decades later, plagued by a rampant and more virulent malignant dyspepsia, Hitler would be responsible for the eviction from Germany of R. Schindler (the founder of modern endoscopy), I. Boas (the founder of gastroenterology) and H. Lamm (the first to transmit an image through glass fibers). The men whose intellectual contributions would serve to elucidate the origins of dyspepsia.

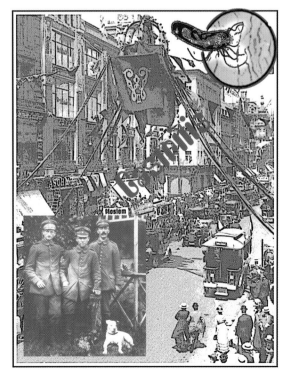

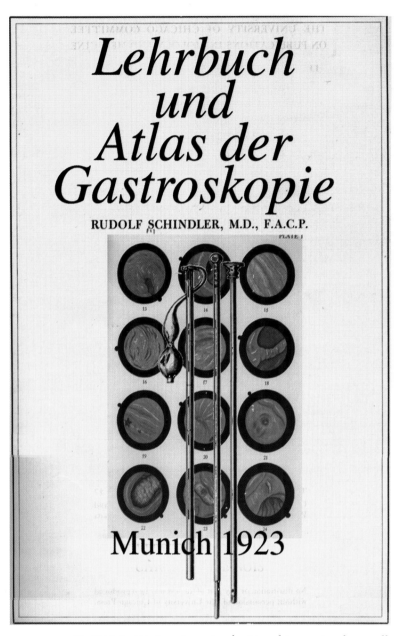

Lehrbuch und Atlas der Gastroskopie

RUDOLF SCHINDLER, M.D., F.A.C.P.

Munich 1923

The *"Lehrbuch und Atlas der Gastroskopie"*, published in 1923 by R.Schindler while working at the Schwabing hospital in Munich, would become both the mantra and lodestone of gastroscopists for the next two decades.

would become his most important clinical assistant and was critical to the development of gastroscopic skills. Indeed, such was her skill with patients, that if Gabriele was unavailable Schindler even in later years would defer endoscopic examination of a patient.

Driven by the belief that gastroscopy would provide a unique diagnostic window to the resolution of gastric disease, Schindler displayed such enthusiasm and commitment to the subject that by 1923, he had already published an atlas of gastroscopy, *"Lehrbuch und Atlas der Gastroskopie"*.

This first and classic contribution to the clinical and diagnostic assessment of the stomach would mark the initiation of his subsequent 45-year focus on demonstrating the utility of gastroscopy. During a long and often tempestuous life Schindler directed his attention to assuring not only the technological improvement of the instruments, but also the development and teaching of appropriate clinical techniques for their usage. He was particularly committed to the concept of clinical scholarship and came early to the recognition of the necessity to obtain detailed documentation of gastroscopic experience for publication and critical evaluation.

At his death in 1968, his exemplary record as a teacher, skilled gastroenterologist and innovator deservedly earned him the sobriquet of "The Father of Gastroscopy." In this context his family played a considerable role. Thus his wife Gabriele was his chief clinical assistant, while his son, Richard, and his daughter, Ursula, were themselves important contributors to his gastroscopy program. Thus Schindler credited Richard at the tender age of 11 as being the first to suggest that adequate anesthesia of the patient's throat might best be achieved by construction of a tube with perforations placed along its length rather than only at its tip. This innovative suggestion allowed for anesthetic spray to be simultaneously delivered throughout the length of the throat instead of simply at the area adjacent to the tip. Richard was also involved in the development of Schindler's slide projection system, while his daughter, Ursula, helped not only in slide shows but also in the typing of manuscripts.

MUNICH 1920

Having acquired a reputation not only as a gastroenterologist of insight but as a skillful gastroscopist, Schindler embarked on what was to become his lifework — the establishment of gastroscopy as a worthy discipline. In particular he was determined that appropriate indications for gastroscopy be determined and that both the instrument and the operator be regarded as safe. The latter concerns reflected the somewhat cavalier approach that had become associated with some of the early proponents of the technique. In 1922 a brush with his colleague, Wilhelm Sternberg, produced an unfortunate incident that highlighted the nature of this problem. In seeking to persuade older and influential physicians of the utility of the technique, Schindler had embarked upon a series of demonstrations. Having successfully demonstrated the use of his rigid instrument to Ernst Sauerbruch, a former student and close friend of Mikulicz, Schindler thereafter refused to appear on the program with Sternberg, whose skills and instrument had given him cause for concern. As Schindler predicted, Sternberg exercised poor judgement in undertaking to endoscope an unsuitable patient and the esophageal tear culminated in mediastinitis and demise of the patient.

The acceptance of gastroscopy in Europe and particular Germany received a severe setback when the highly regarded Munich surgeon, E.F. Sauerbruch (*left*) published an outspoken condemnation (*"Gastroscopy with Deadly Consequences"*) of the procedure (*bottom right*). Sauerbruch had invited Schindler and Sternberg to demonstrate the efficacy of the technique but since Schindler had reservations about both the instrument and skills of his colleague he declined to appear. Undeterred by this rebuff, Sternberg proceeded to attempt endoscopy on a problematic patient culminating in esophageal perforation, mediastinitis and death. As a result Sauerbruch penned a damning indictment of gastroscopy and denounced its clinical utility.

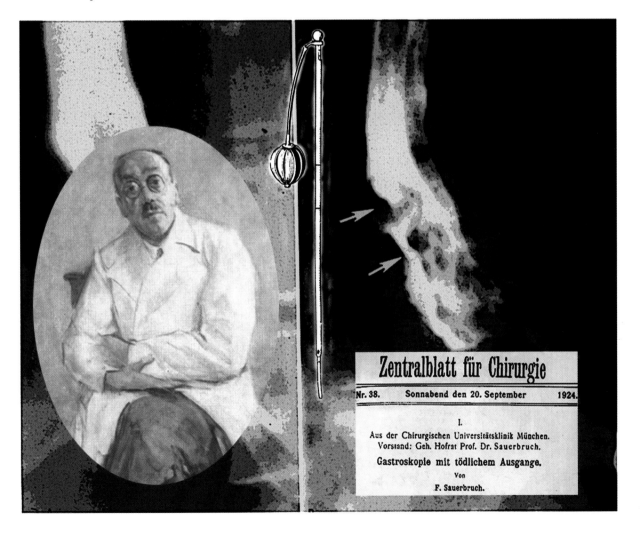

Zentralblatt für Chirurgie

Nr. 38.   Sonnabend den 20. September   1924.

I.

Aus der Chirurgischen Universitätsklinik München.
Vorstand: Geh. Hofrat Prof. Dr. Sauerbruch.

Gastroskopie mit tödlichem Ausgange.

Von

F. Sauerbruch.

The influential and outspoken Sauerbruch, while complimentary of Schindler's technique, seized the opportunity to publish the outcome of the demonstration and widely denounced gastroscopy as a procedure capable of a "deadly outcome." Indeed the significant opposition of an influential surgeon such as Sauerbruch combined with Schindler's belief that gastroscopy should be undertaken in an office setting rather than operating room played a substantial part in diminishing the initial role of surgeons in the development of this technique.

Despite his early success and acclaim it was apparent to Schindler that the potential problem of stomach perforations and esophageal tears with rigid instruments would be the rate-limiting factor in the development of the discipline. This recognition was further amplified by discussions with two American gastroenterologists, Marie Ortmayer and Grant Laing of Chicago, who visited him in 1924 in Munich. Ortmayer and Laing were touring medical centers in Europe and during their sojourn in Vienna serendipitously unearthed a copy of Schindler's "Lehrbuch" in a Vienna bookshop. Impressed with the possibilities contained therein they elected to travel to Munich and on meeting with him to further explore the subject were struck with his knowledge and skill of gastroscopy. This chance meeting was to lead to a subsequent encounter with Walter Palmer, Chairman of the Department of Gastroenterology at the University of Chicago, and the development of a lifelong association.

GEORG WOLF

As a result of his own experience and discussions with others, Schindler became convinced that the resolution of the issue of instrument "flexibility" was the critical variable necessary for the development of successful gastroscopy. Strongly

Georg Wolf (1873-1938) of Berlin was the instrument manufacturer responsible for bringing Rudolf Schindler's dreams of a flexible endoscope to fruition. Although widely reputed for his manufacture of cystoscopic instruments his initial endeavor in designing a flexible gastroscope (*top and bottom insets*) with Sussman (1911) had failed. Despairing of such a possibility, he thereafter limited himself to manufacturing under his imprimatur (*top right and bottom center*) a variety of rigid instruments for Elsner, Hubner and Hohlweg. Schindler and Wolf addressed the problems of the Elsner instrument and by 1923 had redesigned it by adding an air outlet to clear the lens as well as using the rubber tip only as a guide. After introduction the rubber tip was withdrawn and the inner tube and lens inserted.

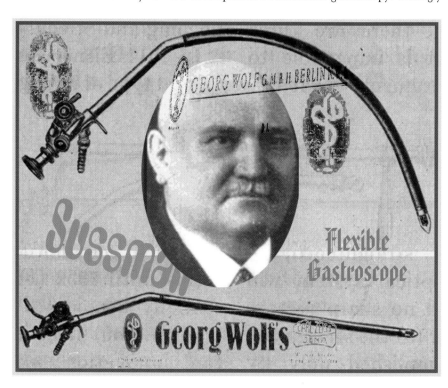

motivated by this concept, he sought out Georg Wolf (1873-1938), the Berlin manufacturer who had initially produced the Sussmann "flexible gastroscope" of 1911. Although Wolf had demonstrated unusual mechanical ingenuity in the actual construction of this device, it had proved unwieldy to use and of little clinical utility.

Wolf's next step was to utilize a fascinating proposal of Michael Hoffman, who in 1911 had reported that vision was not only possible in a linear environment (rigid tube) but could be undertaken under conditions of "curvature" if numerous prisms were inserted into a movable tube. Based on Hoffman's concept, Wolf thereupon constructed a gastroscope with a tip, which could be moved backwards and forwards through an angle of 180° without diminishing the clarity of view. Despite the fact that the visual acuity was considerably improved, this instrument was as clumsy as the Sussmann gastroscope and there was little interest or demand for it from physicians. Wolf thereupon dropped the idea and for the next 15 years confined himself to producing rigid instruments according to modifications provided by Hubner, Hohlweg and Elsner.

The subsequent relationship with Schindler rekindled Wolf's belief in the need for a flexible gastroscope. Together they sought to produce a thin flexible tube whose length and flexibility would not only enable lenses to be mounted in such a fashion that flexion would not interfere with vision, but retain adequate length to comfortably reach the stomach. In order to accommodate these criteria, Wolf produced six gastroscope prototypes between 1928 and 1932. Thus on July 13, 1930 patent #629,590 was awarded to Georg Wolf for the development of the first fully flexible gastroscope, which contained a sequence of lenses screwed to the sides of the tube. A further modification resulted in yet another patent filing and on July 7th, 1932 patent #662,788 was similarly awarded to Georg Wolf for his design of the semi-flexible gastroscope.

The latter model was unique in that it contained lenses, which were displaceable along the interior of the tube following the transmission of an elastic pressure provided by a bronze coil located at the distal end. Thus increasing the tension on the coil allowed the lenses to be pushed against the upper end into a space separating the rigid and flexible segments. Such was the success of this design that the introduction of the instrument resulted in "a rapid, almost explosive, spread of the gastroscopic method." Not unaware of the staggering potential of his device Wolf had within three years successfully applied for and received a U.S. patent for this gastroscope. Thus on March 17, 1935 the U.S. patent # 1,995,196 was awarded for the invention of a semi-flexible gastroscope.

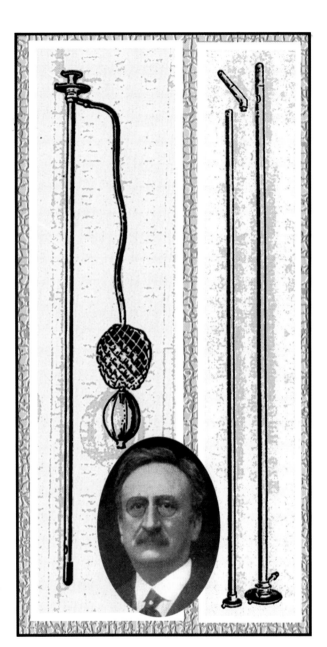

Hans Elsner (*bottom*) of Berlin introduced his model of the rigid endoscope in 1911 and it remained in the words of Schindler "the mother of all instruments until 1932." The instrument was for practical purposes a modification of Theodor Rosenheim's device of 1896, but had been improved by the addition of a rubber tube at the end of the straight tip. Although the lens and light system were incorporated into an inner tube, a critical limitation was that the lens was particularly susceptible to soiling, with consequent poor visibility.

The Lens Problem

Although the mechanical issues of flexibility had to a degree been overcome, the significant obstacle that remained was the maintenance of visual acuity. In particular the precise arrangements of the lenses located in the flexible portion still posed a design issue of considerable magnitude. As early as 1916 Langer of the Berlin optical company, Goertz, had described that "a thick convex lens would transmit a picture through a flexible tube and through exchangeable curves." Although Schindler was initially unaware of this information, Wolf was swift to perceive the application of this observation and utilized the technique in the construction of the flexible gastroscope. Thus the flexible component of the endoscope consisted of six equal elements, each of which contained three spaces with two of the spaces carrying double convex lens and one a simple convex lens, resulting in a total of 31 lenses. Each space was 15mm apart and articulated with the adjacent one by a ball and socket joint. Thus in the 24cm of the flexible area, the six elements each produced a real image in its last focal plane that remained intact when the entire system was bent into an arch of up to 34°. The entire gastroscope consisted of 51 opti-

The problem of maintaining adequate visibility in a flexible system was a novel difficulty for optical engineers, who had previously dealt only with rigid systems such as telescopes and microscopes. The added issue was the need to not only miniaturize the components, but also render the housing absolutely waterproof since any moisture altered the transmission characteristics of the image. J.H. Hett successfully resolved the problem by providing specific criteria for a multiple flexible lens system of 51 optical elements (US patent issued Feb 16, 1949). As a result of this advance the angle of flexion could be increased to 55° without any significant image distortion or loss.

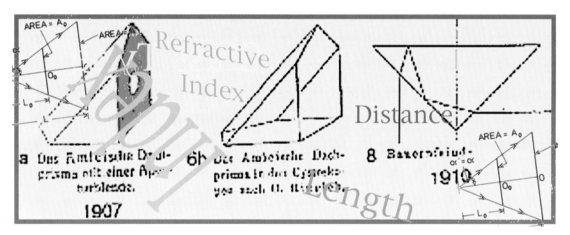

cal elements and it was the critical spacing of the lenses that would become the rate-limiting factor in determining the evolution of gastroscopy up until the advent of fiber optic technology. The mathematical proof and raw diagrams delineating the precise lens details (distances, thickness, glass type, refractive index, etc) required for each lens in the flexible section was subsequently the subject of a detailed patent specification submitted to the U.S. patent office by J. H. Hett on February 16, 1949. These modifications allowed for the amplification of the original Wolf design in that the angle to which the instrument could be bent could now be increased to 55° prior to loss of image.

Some American controversy in regard to the design of the flexible optic system for the gastroscope arose from the association of Samuel Weiss of New York with Schindler and Wolf. An innovative physician, Weiss had graduated from Long Island Medical College in 1907 and by 1914 had turned his attention to gastroenterology and becoming one of the first physicians in New York to install an X-ray machine in his office. He subsequently became the editor of the *American Journal of Gastroenterology*, which position he held for 33 years with considerable acclaim. Having spent some time with Schindler in Munich, he thereafter campaigned vigorously in an attempt

Samuel Weiss of New York (1914) was an early American pioneer of endoscopy. As editor of the American Journal of Gastroenterology for 33 years and a trainee of Schindler he became an influential voice in the field of gastroscopy.

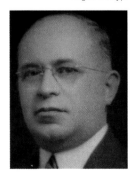

to persuade American physicians to accept gastroscopy.

Not only did he publish a paper entitled "A New Gastroscope", but he also invested considerable time and effort on the design problems of the flexible optical system. Having initially visited Schindler in 1925, he subsequently returned in 1927 with his own sketches relating to the design of a new gastroscope. Schindler advised him to discuss his plans with Georg Wolf and as a result Weiss met with Wolf and left him copies of this proposed contrivance. Some months later Wolf declined by letter to further pursue the proposal, indicating that he considered the designs of Weiss to be impractical in regard to the construction of a gastric endoscope. The subsequent publication and patent filing of Wolf's gastroscope dismayed Weiss, who was adamant in the belief that his designs had been incorporated into the new instrument without appro-

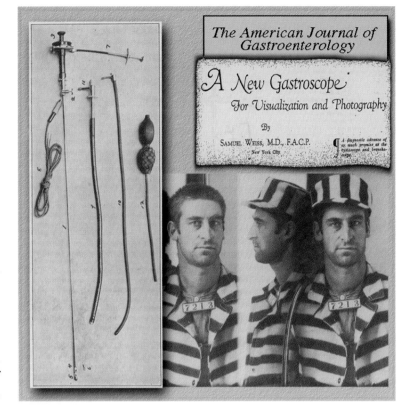

priate acknowledgement. Weiss, however, was undaunted in his support of gastroscopy and such was his enthusiasm in the promotion of the instrument and its clinical utility that in 1932 he demonstrated the use of the rigid gastroscope on no less than six prisoners at Sing Sing State Penitentiary in Ossining, New York!

S. Weiss of New York City had visited Schindler in Munich on a number of occasions with a view to perfecting his gastroscopic skills. In 1927 he submitted his own gastroscope design to Georg Wolf, who rejected the proposals as impractical. The subsequent patent filing by Wolf upset Weiss, who believed that his ideas had been utilized but not acknowledged. Nevertheless Weiss remained an ardent practitioner of gastroscopy and played a significant role in popularizing the use of the instrument (*left*) by both publications (*top right*) and practical presentations. Such was his enthusiasm for the technique that in 1932 he even traveled to Sing Sing State penitentiary in Ossining, NY, where he examined six prisoners to demonstrate the efficacy and safety of the technique. The matter of the manner in which informed consent for this exercise was obtained is still a source of debate.

THE CHICAGO TRANSFER

Despite the emancipated intellectual environment of Germany, the advent of political instability and egregious racism would temporally engulf the career of Rudolf Schindler in a penumbra of potentially numinous doom. The advent of Hitler and the Brown Shirts generated a subversive environment in which even the most innocent found themselves the victims of the most debased. Thus shortly after introduction of the semi-flexible gastroscope and his recognition as physician of international consequence, Schindler was denounced to the "authorities" by his housekeeper. Allegedly angry at the termination of her employment she countered by claiming that Schindler was a subversive responsible for the perpetration of crimes against innocent German citizens. As the son of a Jewish father and a Lutheran mother, Schindler was considered "tainted" and the Nazis accused him of being an enemy of the State. Utilizing the age-old euphemism for politically sanctioned thuggery, he was thereupon placed in "protective custody" in no less salubrious an environment than Dachau. The explanation was that a full investigation of the charges that had been made against him was required and that such custody was simply to protect him in order that "the righteously indignant citizens of Munich would not do harm to him." Clearly the problems faced by endoscopy, namely rigidity and vision, were endemic to the politics of the time. Aware that protective custody of this type was often associated with inexplicable accidents and disappearances, his wife Gabriele exerted considerable efforts in an attempt to obtain his release. Nevertheless, despite the obvious international scandal that would follow his "disappearance", six months were to elapse before Schindler would be able to leave the country. Fortunately Marie Ortmayer supported his request for the opportunity to join the staff of the University of Chicago and obtained support from donors to subsidize such an appointment. Thus in 1934 Schindler and his family departed Nazi Germany and he assumed an appointment as visiting professor at the University of Chicago under the Chairmanship of Walter Palmer. Financial subsidy for this venture was provided by George Baehr, Chairman of the Refugee Physician's Fund and other Chicago physicians. Of particular benefit was the support provided by Mrs. C. Morse and Mrs. M. Fisher. Indeed both had a decade earlier provided fiscal support to cover the costs of the publication of the color plates contained in Schindler's first publication, "*The Atlas of Gastroscopy*".

THE NEW WORLD

Schindler was well received in Chicago not only as a surviving victim of persecution but as a substantial clinician and a gastroenterologist of great experience and skill. In addition, having trained over 300 physicians in the use of both the rigid and semi-flexible instrument, he was well versed in the arts of gastroscopy. Thus warmly supported by his family and friends, as well as embraced by respectful colleagues and a politically emancipated environment, Schindler soon regained his

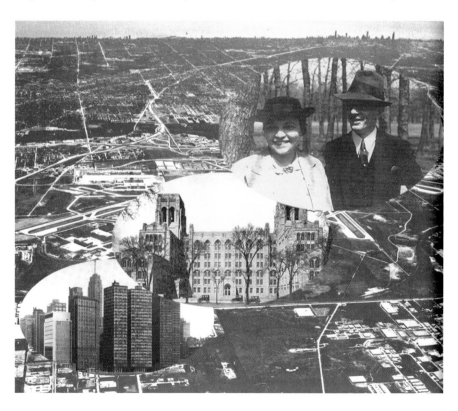

Gabriele and Rudolf Schindler (*top right*) arrived with their two children Richard and Ursula in Chicago in the summer of 1934. Rudolf joined Walter L. Palmer, Joseph B. Kirsner and Marie Ortmayer at the Gastrointestinal Unit of the University of Chicago and soon established a busy gastroscopic practice. A dynamic individual of considerable versatility and skill, Schindler had within three years translated and published his book on gastroscopy, earned the reputation of being a "masterful teacher".

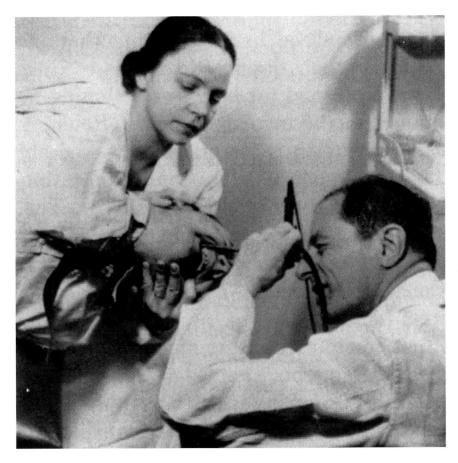

Mrs. Gabriele Schindler holding the head of a patient while her husband performs an upper gastro intestinal endoscopy (circa 1940). Although not medically trained, Schindler regarded her expert assistance as paramount to the success of any gastroscopic procedure. Indeed her unavailability for any reason would prompt him to instantly cancel all scheduled patients. An indefatigable worker and rigid taskmaster, Schindler was capable of performing more than 10 gastroscopies every 2.5 hours. Thus by 1947 he had personally examined 2,500 patients with gastritis and published a definitive monograph on the subject. So effective was the husband and wife team that the Chicago clinic was soon overwhelmed with visiting physicians seeking to learn the methodology of the master. Indeed such was the national interest that by 1941 Schindler had recognized the need for a formal gastroscopic organization and taken steps to establish a society.

highly productive work ethic. As such he became responsible for a daily private clinic at the Billings Hospital and continued to undertake gastroscopy as well as to write productively. Palmer provided considerable support in helping the German speaking Schindler convert to facile English and Marie Ortmayer remained an important professional and personal friend. Gabriele amplified her role as his professional assistant and became adept at both preparing his patients for gastroscopy as well as managing them during and after the procedure. Indeed a number of accounts of this time recall how critical Gabriele was in ensuring Schindler's successful performance of gastroscopy. Her empathic persona and calm gravity as well as technical skills were important both for reassuring patients as well as for maintaining the critical positioning of the head during the endoscopic procedure.

Nevertheless the environment was not entirely conducive to relaxation and success. The milieu of Chicago in the 1930s and 1940s differed somewhat from that of the sophistication of Munich. Furthermore, concerns of territorial primacy and imperative relating to the influx of foreign-trained physicians to America also provided for some discomfort. Similarly, basic commercial concerns were raised by the incumbents and trade issues involving client base and remuneration also evolved from the influx of numerous skilled European physicians. Thus gratitude for professional and personal salvation was often diluted or even obscured in the anxiety and pressure generated by different work attitudes and the lack of familiar support systems. Nevertheless, despite the obstacles provided by the necessity of obtaining U.S. citizenship and the need to secure acceptable medical accreditation, Schindler exceeded

78

Marie Ortmayer had first met Schindler in Munich in 1927. Their friendship and mutual professional appreciation were to prove felicitous in that Ortmayer played a prominent role in securing a position and support for Schindler in Chicago as the rising tide of German political unrest threatened his safety. Ortmayer was actively involved in Schindler's work and her major contributions to the field of gastroscopy were appropriately recognized in 1954 on her election as the first female president of the American Gastroscopic Society.

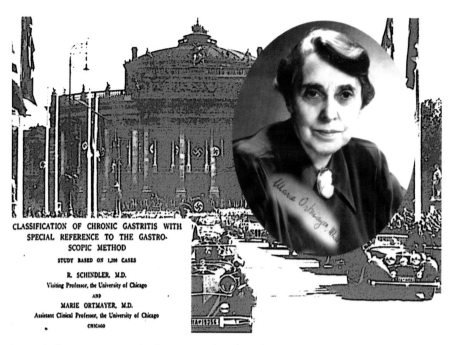

CLASSIFICATION OF CHRONIC GASTRITIS WITH SPECIAL REFERENCE TO THE GASTRO-SCOPIC METHOD

STUDY BASED ON 1,200 CASES

R. SCHINDLER, M.D.
Visiting Professor, the University of Chicago
AND
MARIE ORTMAYER, M.D.
Assistant Clinical Professor, the University of Chicago
CHICAGO

Walter Lincoln Palmer (c. 1937), Chief of the Gastrointestinal Unit at the University of Chicago. An early friend and strong supporter of Schindler, their relationship rapidly deteriorated. Having repudiated Schindler's views on gastritis, Palmer declined to support his tenure and in 1943 Schindler departed to Los Angeles.

beyond all expectations at both a personal and professional level. Although the subliminal and often overt discrimination by American physicians against the medical refugees of this time produced some difficulties, Schindler's name would soon become a household word and his contributions to gastroscopy become both nationally and internationally recognized. In this respect a great debt of gratitude is owed to the clinical perspicuity and intellectual and moral generosity of Marie Ortmayer. Without her and her supporters it is likely that the rightful advent of gastroscopy might not only have been significantly delayed but Schindler like Ismar Boas, the founder of gastroenterology, would have perished as a victim of the Holocaust.

TWILIGHT DAYS

Unfortunately in 1943, little less than a decade after his triumphal arrival, Schindler departed Chicago, having been ignominiously refused tenure. This unfortunate situation reflected the culmination of some years of personal and professional tension emanating both from Schindler's autocratic European style and his dogmatic assertions concerning gastritis that were decried by the Chairman, Walter Palmer. Schindler and Palmer had long nourished a mutual animus regarding Schindler's fascination with the topic of gastritis. The publication in 1942 by Palmer of a paper entitled *"The Stomach and Military Service"*, which

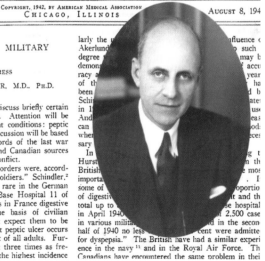

The Journal of the American Medical Association

Published Under the Auspices of the Board of Trustees

VOL. 119, No. 15 | COPYRIGHT, 1942, BY AMERICAN MEDICAL ASSOCIATION CHICAGO, ILLINOIS | AUGUST 8, 194

THE STOMACH AND MILITARY SERVICE

CHAIRMAN'S ADDRESS

WALTER LINCOLN PALMER, M.D., PH.D.
CHICAGO

My purpose in this paper is to discuss briefly certain military aspects of gastric disease. Attention will be centered on the two most frequent conditions: peptic ulcer and chronic gastritis. The discussion will be based on civilian experience, on the records of the last war and on the reports from British and Canadian sources since the outbreak of the present conflict.

In the first world war gastric disorders were, according to Hurst,[1] rather "rare among soldiers." Schindler,[2] however, states that they were not rare in the German army, and Dick[3] recalls that in Base Hospital 11 of the American Expeditionary Forces in France digestive disorders were common. On the basis of civilian experience, indeed, one would not expect them to be rare. Autopsy studies indicate that peptic ulcer occurs at some time in at least 12 per cent of all adults. Furthermore, the lesion appears about three times as frequently in males as in females, and the highest incidence

larly the ... Akerlund ... degree ... demons ... racy a ... of th ... been ... Schi ... in 1 ... And ... can ... whe ... sary ... In ... Hurst ... British ... importa ... some of ... of digestiv ... total up to ... in April 1940 ... in various milita ... half of 1940 no less ... for dyspepsia." The British have had a similar experience in the navy[11] and in the Royal Air Force. Th Canadians have encountered the same problem in thei disparaged the limited evidence supporting Schindler's theories of gastritis, provided the final denouement to this already tenuous relationship. Dissatisfied with Palmer's feelings and incensed at the perceived lack of support, Schindler in 1943 departed for Los Angeles and the College of Medical Evangelists, now known as the Loma Linda University. Ensconced in the salubrious environment of Southern California he continued his practice at the College, while continuing to provide professional support for instrument corporations as well as the Veterans Administration medical system and a number of private clinics. Approaching the retirement age and still interested in new experiences, Schindler in 1958 accepted an appointment as Professor of Medicine at the University of Minas Gerais in Belo Horizonte, Brazil. Rapidly mastering the Brazilian language he successfully taught there for two years until the failing health of Gabriele forced his return to the United States in 1960. Thereafter he became a consultant at the Long Beach Veterans Administration Hospital until 1964, when upon the demise of Gabriele he once again sought the familiar pastures of his youth. In 1965 Schindler remarried an old friend of his Munich days, Mary Koch, and retired to Munich where he died in 1968.

During his lifetime Schindler had produced more than 170 manuscripts and 5 books, including the seminal *"Lehrbuch"* of 1923. In 1937 he published his classic monograph on gastroscopy and in 1947 a controversial publication on gastritis. In 1957 he produced the widely accepted *"Synopsis of Gastroenterology"*, which detailed not only the contributions of endoscopy, but placed Schindler's own personal views on the subject in perspective. In this respect he recognized the special merit of gastroscopy in the early detection of gastric disease, but fully accepted the necessity for the interface between both radiology and gastroscopy in the accurate and early diagnosis of stomach disease.

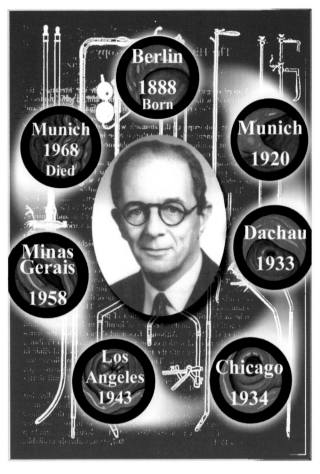

Rudolf Schindler (1888–1968).

EPITAPH

A brilliant man possessed of a formidable intellect and occasionally irascible nature, Schindler was an intriguing amalgam of sophistication, high intellect and exotic eclecticism. A product of two cultures and two centuries, he saw and dared what few had done before. Resilient, innovative, consumed by curiosity and gifted with extraordinary insight and perspicuity, he strove and succeeded in extending the boundaries of diagnosis. None who worked with him would ever forget him and whether he engendered love, admiration or sometimes even frustration, his outstanding contributions would forever change the way physicians viewed *le milieu interieur*. A worthy first president of the American Gastroscopic Club, Schindler might rightfully claim, as did Newton of Hooke, "that I saw further by standing on the shoulders of the giants who had gone before me."

CHAPTER 2 | *American Gastroscopy*

ON HIS ARRIVAL in the United States, American gastroscopy, though in its infancy, had nevertheless acquired some significant proponents. These included Chevalier Jackson of Philadelphia, John C. Hemmeter of Baltimore, Edward B. Benedict of Boston as well as Elihu Katz, Max Einhorn, Samuel Weiss and Henry Harrington Janeway of New York.

Of particular interest are the contributions of Frederick C. Herrick of Cleveland, who in 1911 had described a gastroscope that could be introduced directly into the stomach via the abdominal incision during surgery. In reality this was no more than a modified cystoscope which he utilized to locate the site of the ulcer and thus claimed benefit in restricting the size of the incision into the stomach. His observations were recorded in the *Cleveland Medical Journal* of 1911 under the title of "*Profuse Recurrent Gastric Hemorrhage with the Report of Cases and a description of an Instrument of viewing the Gastric Interior at operation*". Despite such early innovation and considerable enthusiasm, the pace of development in American was not as rapid as might have been anticipated. John Hemmeter of Johns Hopkins Hospital had commented as early as 1897 in "*Diseases of the Stomach*" (the first comprehensive American text on the subject) that gastroscopy "had an undoubted future development as a diagnostic aid." Unfortunately, in spite of such optimistic perspicuity, at his death in 1931 such glowing predictions regarding gastroscopy had failed to achieve reality in Baltimore.

Nevertheless by 1934 the Wolf-Schindler gastroscope was already in use at Baltimore having been brought there by James L. Borland. Although Borland subsequently moved to Jacksonville, Florida, John T. Howard, E. B. Freeman and Moses Paulson of the Johns Hopkins Hospital had also acquired an instrument and trials to evaluate the procedure were in soon in place. Such efforts were mostly due to the enthusiasm of Ball, who had undertaken a post-graduate training course in endoscopy in Philadelphia with Chevalier Jackson and transmitted his enthusiasm for the subject of gastroscopy to his colleagues.

Jackson's interest in examination of the esophagus and stomach stemmed from his success at examining the trachea and bronchi with a rigid instrument containing no lenses. An outspoken individual of great clinical skill and experience, Jackson was an ardent advocate of the safety of the open tube gastroscope. Both he and his colleague, Benjamin Thomas, believed firmly and vigorously maintained, that the attempts to modify cystoscope construction with lenses for gastroscopy had been responsible for the inordinate delay in enabling the design of a safe gastroscope. Impervious to such Philadelphian commentary, Janeway and Green of New York worked tenaciously to publish a report in 1911 documenting 50 successful gastroscopies and adumbrated on the obvious advantage of the methodology in identifying gastric carcinoma at an early stage. In reality it seems apparent that many different physicians, each in their own unique fashion, sought to promote gastroscopy, though none had the experience and obsession of Schindler.

Henry H. Janeway of New York. A surgeon of diverse skills and immense productivity, Janeway addressed almost every contemporary issue with rigor and zeal. His contributions to establishing the efficacy of gastroscopy were substantial and as early as 1911 he had in collaboration with Nathan Green advocated the use of gastroscopy in the early diagnosis of gastric neoplasia.

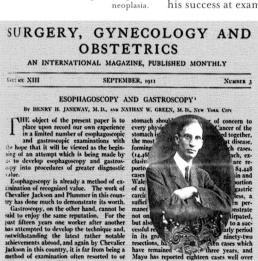

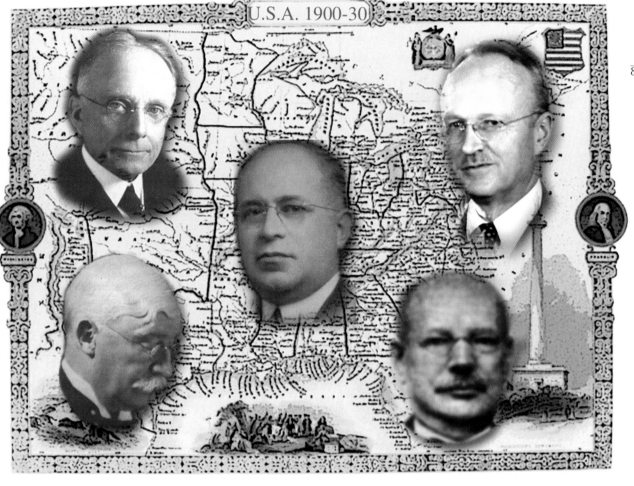

U.S.A. 1900-30

Probably the most enthusiastic of the American endoscopists was Edward Benedict of Boston. By early 1933 Benedict had become aware of the new Schindler flexible gastroscope and had obtained the support of his mentors at the Massachusetts General Hospital, Chester Jones and Edward Churchill, to undertake its usage. A Wolf-Schindler instrument had been acquired for trial use, courtesy of Carl Zeiss of Jena, the maker of the optics for the instrument, and on April 6, 1933 Benedict and Jones undertook the first examination with it. Benedict reported his very positive first experience: "...our first patient was a man who later proved to have a gastric lymphoma. We did not make the diagnosis, needless to say, on our first gastroscopic attempt. In fact I believe we could do it now only with gastroscopic biopsy. (Benedict would become a pioneer and proponent of gastroscopic biopsy). Anyway, from then on my work in gastroscopy was started: Dr. Churchill suggested that I add bronchoscopy and esophagoscopy and Dr. Allen suggested peritoneoscopy too. So I gave up general surgery altogether and devoted myself entirely to endoscopy." Determined to become an expert he visited the eminent French gastroscopist, Moutier, and rapidly became familiar with the use of the gastroscope. Thus by 1934 Benedict had performed 75 gastroscopies with the Wolf-Schindler instrument and his skill and expertise were such that they rivaled those of Schindler. Despite his location within a bastion of Boston conservatism, Benedict was destined to become not only a devotee

The Doyens of American Gastroscopy 1900-1930. Chevalier Jackson of Philadelphia (top left) was an otolaryngologist and esophagoscopist of extraordinary skill. His ability to extract foreign bodies from the esophagus became legendary and the collection is currently housed at the Mutter Museum in Philadelphia. Edward Benedict of Boston (top right) was an astute surgeon whose prescience enabled him to grasp the possibilities of gastroscopy and laparoscopy. Max Einhorn of New York (bottom right) was revered as a clinician, scholar and innovative thinker. In attestation of his contributions a sculptured plaque at Lennox Hill Hospital in NYC depicts him with I. Boas and A. Kussmaul. John Hemmeter of Baltimore (bottom left) produced a textbook "Diseases of the Stomach" that attained biblical status. Samuel Weiss (center) of New York was editor of the American Journal of Gastroenterology for more than three decades and an ardent supporter of gastroscopy.

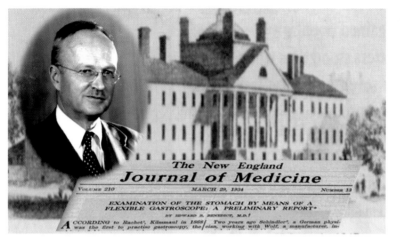

The New England
Journal of Medicine

VOLUME 210   MARCH 29, 1934   NUMBER 13

EXAMINATION OF THE STOMACH BY MEANS OF A
FLEXIBLE GASTROSCOPE: A PRELIMINARY REPORT*

BY EDWARD B. BENEDICT, M.D.!

ACCORDING to Rachet¹, Küssmaul in 1868 | Two years ago Schindler², a German physi-
was the first to practise gastroscopy, the | cian, working with Wolf, a manufacturer, in-

Edward Benedict of Boston
(*top left*) was one of the most
enthusiastic of the American
endoscopists. Having
obtained the support of his
mentors Chester Jones and
Edward Churchill at the
Massachusetts General
Hospital (*center*), to undertake
gastroscopy he acquired a
Wolf-Schindler instrument
for trial use, courtesy of Carl
Zeiss of Jena (the maker of
the optics for the
instrument). On April 6
1933 Benedict and Jones
undertook the first
examination. Benedict
reported his very positive first
experience, "our first patient
was a man who later proved to
have a gastric lymphoma. We
did not make the diagnosis,
needless to say, on our first
gastroscopic attempt. In fact I
believe we could do it now
only with gastroscopic
biopsy." (Benedict would
subsequently become a
pioneer and avid proponent
of gastroscopic biopsy).
Determined to attain
expertise, he visited the
eminent French
gastroscopist, Moutier, in
Paris and rapidly became
adept. In 1934 Benedict
published his experience with
75 gastroscopies (*bottom*) using
the Wolf-Schindler
instrument and established
his position as an expert in
the evolving field. Despite his
location within a bastion of
Boston conservatism,
Benedict was destined to
become a prophet of the
future efficacy of gastroscopy
and would succeed Schindler
to become the second
president of the American
Gastroscopic Club.

and innovator, but also a prophet of the future efficacy of gastroscopy.

Since Benedict was a surgeon, he was particularly interested in the use of the technique to obtain tissue and by 1948 had developed an operating gastroscope for the acquisition of gastric tissue in conjunction with the American Cystoscope Makers Corporation. In this endeavor Schindler initially provided considerable support since he believed that the use of laparotomy and exploratory surgery were unduly dangerous for the acquisition of biopsy material.

A particular source of concern at this time in the United States was the incidence of esophageal and gastric perforation. So serious was this consideration that in 1936 activity was informally suspended in Schindler's clinic for about six months while the cause of the perforations was investigated. Palmer believed that the esophagus was the problem and suggested that Schindler leave its evaluation to ear, nose, and throat specialists while concentrating on the stomach. Schindler, however, determined after careful experimental measurements conducted upon cadaver stomachs that the perforations of the posterior wall depended upon the type of tip used. He determined that an elongated rubber tip was superior in protecting the stomach and caused less damage than a rounded sponge or the shorter rubber tip previously used. With his characteristic zeal Schindler thereafter in 1940 conducted a poll of sixty American gastroscopists and determined that out of 22,351 gastroscopies only 8 perforations of the stomach had occurred with one fatality (a mortality of .004%).

CAMERON AND STREIFENEDER

Accustomed as he was to working with Georg Wolf of Berlin, one of Schindler's challenges upon moving to the United States was to identify a technical expert of similar capabilities. In this respect William J. Cameron, the founder of the Cameron Surgical Company of Chicago and one of the largest manufacturers of illuminated medical instruments in the world, adequately fitted the bill. Cameron, a Canadian immigrant with a degree in pharmacy, had begun his business by designing and developing a dental light used for the purpose of defining gum pyorrhea. His interest in working with Schindler was particularly piqued by the opportunity to provide gastroscopes to American physicians since the supply of German endoscopes had been curtailed by the advent of the World War II. Thus by 1940 an improved Cameron gastroscope had been designed and was freely available in the marketplace. Its improvements included a slightly reduced angle of vision (from 50° to 45°) with a consequent increase in magnification and a reduced depth of focus with the result that the objective could be made wider and more light could enter the cavity thus creating a brighter image. In addition more flexible material had been introduced to replace the bronze spiral used to hold the lenses in place in the flexible portion and the casing of the optical system had been placed in a bonded rubber coating rather than the clumsy rubber hose that had been formerly used. Embedding the electric wire in this rubber layer to obviate any likelihood of short circuit or shock if the patient inadvertently bit the tube provided a further innovation.

To the delight of the meticulous Schindler the company staff included an excellent technician, Louis Streifeneder, who was adept and quick to respond to Schindler's suggestions regarding instrument modification. Fanatic about the details of construction, Schindler had required that the initial Wolf-Schindler gastroscope be revised five times. Indeed the substantial mutual regard shared by the two was such that their association would last for more than three decades and result in a significant amplification of the original Wolf-Schindler gastroscope design. An example of Streifeneder's skill was provided by an incident that occurred shortly after Schindler's departure from the University of Chicago involving a number of esophageal perforations that occurred over a short period of time at the Billings Clinic. While such events sometimes reflected poor technique, in many instances the rapidly evolving technology of the instrument was at fault. In this circumstance Louis Streifeneder, who had become a close collaborator of Schindler, determined that a harder and less pliant rubber had mistakenly replaced the rubber of the instrument tip. Since all were aware that the tip was the critical feature in most instances of penetration, much debate had taken place between Schindler, the instrument makers and his colleagues relating to the design (pointed or blunt) and material (metal or rubber) of the tip. Similarly it was Streifeneder who suggested that constructing the lenses out of a lighter flint glass would correct the blue halo that consistently formed around the image when the endoscope was bent more than 30°.

The introduction of the glass lenses of lower lead content resulted in a marked improvement of the image and the innovative Streifeneder subsequently became the founder and director of the Eder Company. In this capacity Streifeneder was influential in introducing numerous modifications (the development of a metal bullet tip for the endoscope, an omni angle movable mirror at the tip, a significantly reduced tube diameter, lens design) to a wide variety of endoscopes including bronchoscopes, cystoscopes, peritoneoscopes, laparoscopes and gastroscopes.

Unfortunately the close relationship with Streifeneder suffered after Schindler's departure from Chicago and in 1945 Schindler arranged for a company that produced picture frames (Metro Tech) to produce a gastroscope made to his own specifications. A particular advantage of the Metro Tech instrument was the use of coated lenses that reduced light absorption and produced a more effective image. Having utilized this proprietary instrument for three years in more than 1000 gastroscopies without any repairs Schindler was of the belief that the Metro Tech instrument was superior to the Eder gastroscope and proposed a formal comparative evaluation. Fortunately their previous mutual regard prevailed and Streifeneder successfully dissuaded him from pursuing this course. Perhaps as a consequence of these events the Metro Tech Instrument Corporation was purchased by the Cameron Surgical Instruments Company

William J. Cameron of the Cameron Surgical Company. Although Cameron (right) had originally trained as a pharmacist he had established a corporation (American Surgical Specialty Company, 1915) that produced illuminated medical instruments. Cameron agreed to work with Schindler and the first flexible gastroscope made in the USA, the Cameron Schindler Endoscope, was produced in 1940. A subsequent model the Flexible Omni Angle Gastroscope (1943) carried a mirror instead of a prism and enabled the endoscopist to view the stomach by moving the mirror and not the instrument itself. Streifeneder, a brilliant technician of the Cameron Company, worked closely with Schindler in perfecting these designs and subsequently played a critical role in the development of instruments by establishing his own facility, the Eder Corporation. Such was the passion which Streifeneder brought to his work, that when gastroscoped by Schindler to evaluate his dyspepsia he noted the stiffness of the brass coil and modified it forthwith.

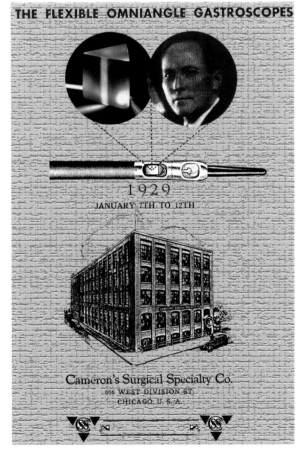

THE FLEXIBLE OMNIANGLE GASTROSCOPES

1929
JANUARY 7TH TO 12TH

Cameron's Surgical Specialty Co.
666 WEST DIVISION ST.
CHICAGO, U. S. A.

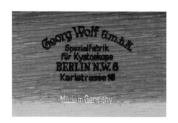

The development of endoscopic instruments was dependent upon a close collaboration between physicians and engineering corporations. In Germany the company of Georg Wolf (*top*) had played a critical role, but after Schindler relocated to Chicago a number of other instrument makers became involved, including the Cameron Co., the Eder instrument Co., Metro Tech and American Cystoscopic Manufacturers Inc.

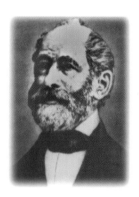

Carl Zeiss (1816-88), founder of the Carl Zeiss Company in 1846. Zeiss was an important supplier of lenses for the early endoscopes.

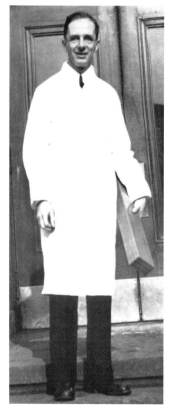

Rudolf Schindler (Chicago c.1937) carrying his gastroscope case. Apart from his endoscopic skills, Schindler was an avid philatelist, conchophile, salamanderphile, Naval historian, Culbertson bridge adept, consummate musician and polylinguist.

in 1959 and production terminated. As a result the Eder instrument became the primary gastroscope in the marketplace and would remain so for a further 15 years until the introduction and development of the fiber optic gastroscope rendered it obsolete. Despite their early differences of opinion, Schindler in 1966 publicly acknowledged that the Eder gastroscope manufactured by Streifeneder's company was the most satisfactory of the standard instruments currently available.

THE FINAL LEGACY

It is worth emphasizing that while Schindler was engrossed in details of the technical design of the endoscope, he was in addition a great proponent of appropriate training and the development of technique. In particular Schindler was a strong advocate of the introduction of a formal education in gastroscopy and insisted that individuals trained in the discipline be regarded as clinicians and gastroenterologists primarily lest they be regarded as only gastroscopists or "mere technicians." In this endeavor he went to great lengths to promote teaching and education in the area of gastroscopy and sought to embrace his colleagues and secure their support in this venture. As a result on November 9th, 1941 in Chicago, Schindler organized at his own apartment the first meeting of those interested in gastroscopy. Although a more detailed account of this seminal meeting may be found elsewhere in this book, a brief description is appropriate at this point. In essence Schindler with a group of like-minded colleagues founded the American Gastroscopic Club with a view to establishing the participation and collaboration of those individuals interested in the advancement of gastroscopy. As the first president and one of its 17 charter members, Schindler thereafter played a significant role in shaping the constitution of this novel club, which included among its objectives the advancement of gastroscopy and gastroscopic diagnosis as well as the development of its relationship to other clinical methods.

The founding group was unanimous in discouraging the commercialization of the gastroscopic method and held that the maintenance of not only high technical quality of the instruments, but the importance of education and the dissemination of information were of paramount concern. Given the extraordinary subsequent success of the endeavor it is of interest to note that the members at this time believed that the group might not function for more than a decade and indeed planned and accepted relatively early apoptotic dissolution of the group. Fortunately their pessimism in this regard has remained unfulfilled and the chrysalis evolved in 1946 into the American Gastroscopic Society and by 1961 had undergone a metamorphosis into the American Society for Gastrointestinal Endoscopy. As such it has more than fulfilled the dreams of its original founding members.

Broadening the Horizon | CHAPTER 3

ESOPHAGOSCOPES OF THE SEMI-FLEXIBLE ERA

Prior to 1940 esophagoscopy had been mainly practiced by individuals who were either involved in bronchoscopy or otolaryngology. Esophagoscopy in fact fell into somewhat of a no man's land since laryngologists, who were usually surgeons and had little knowledge of the upper gastrointestinal tract, mostly practiced it. Those gastroenterologists who were interested in the esophagus were neither trained in surgery nor possessed of any familiarity with introduction of the rigid instruments currently available. However by the late 1940s, a number of semi-flexible devices had been introduced by Boros, Schindler and Hufford, which enabled gastrointestinal endoscopists to enter the field of esophagoscopy.

In June 1947 at the American Medical Association meeting in Atlantic City, NJ, Edwin Boros introduced the device he termed a "flexible esophagogastroscope." Its design to a large extent reflected the original rigid esophagoscope of Chevalier Jackson and despite being termed flexible, did not really meet such criteria. Boros had designed an instrument with a soft pliant tip of spiral coiled metal which since it was somewhat flexible facilitated insertion much as for the semi-flexible original Schindler gastroscope. Having safely introduced the instrument into the esophagus, it was straightened by a metal rod and thereafter a separate light carrier inserted. Within a year of the presentation of his device, Boros claimed to have undertaken "safe, easy, successful esophagoscopies in

The study of the esophagus has proved almost as frustrating as attempts to understand its origin and function. Variously known as the *ysofagus, isofagus, hysophagus, oisophagus* and *ysophague,* it has confounded men from the time of Aristotle to Barrett. The former considered the esophagus to have acquired its name from "its length and its narrowness", but according to its elements it ought to mean *'eater of osiers'*; This derivation seems inept unless it refers to the use of osiers as primitive sounds. The Byzantine Scholiast, Oppian, considered it as derived from *I carry* and *to eat,* which is plausible in the sense of the meaning *"eating (something)".* Although P. Fletcher (1633) disregarded such debate and regarded it quite simply as a "meat pipe conveying meats and drinks to the stomach". Given this confusion, the esophagus was mostly of interest to early physicians as a reservoir for foreign bodies. Despite the wide variety of instruments that had been variously developed (and discarded) for the examination of the stomach, by the turn of the 19th century the esophagus had become a virtual "no man's land". Generally regarded as the province of the otolaryngologist, no one was certain as to how best to examine it, few dared to operate on it and its perforation was feared by all.

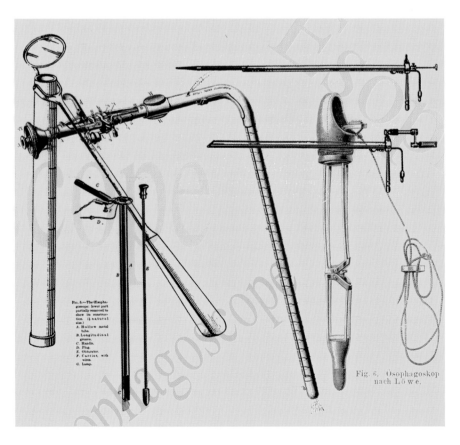

Fig. 6. Osophagoskop nach Löwe.

86

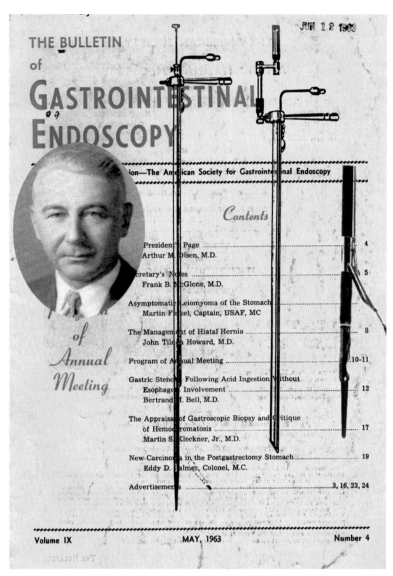

THE BULLETIN
of
GASTROINTESTINAL
ENDOSCOPY

JUN 1 2 1963

ion—The American Society for Gastrointestinal Endoscopy

Contents

President's Page 4
Arthur M. Olsen, M.D.

Secretary's Notes 5
Frank B. McGlone, M.D.

Asymptomatic Leiomyoma of the Stomach
Martin Finkel, Captain, USAF, MC

The Management of Hiatal Hernia 8
John Tilden Howard, M.D.

Program of Annual Meeting 10-11

Gastric Stenosis Following Acid Ingestion Without
Esophageal Involvement 12
Bertrand M. Bell, M.D.

The Appraisal of Gastroscopic Biopsy and Critique
of Hemochromatosis 17
Martin S. Kleckner, Jr., M.D.

New Carcinoma in the Postgastrectomy Stomach ... 19
Eddy D. Palmer, Colonel, M.C.

Advertisements 3, 16, 23, 24

Volume IX   MAY, 1963   Number 4

A. Ray Hufford (*left*) had experimented for a number of years with a variety of optical systems and obturators in a rigid esophagoscope. Having developed a prototype in 1946 he collaborated with Louis Streifeneder of the Eder Instrument Co. and in 1949 the Eder-Hufford esophagoscope was introduced. The device on the left is the outer tube with its obturator and light carrier and in the center is the esophagoscope with the obturator removed and the telescope attached. Not only could the interior of the esophagus be adequately visualized but also biopsies acquired with instruments such as the Kenamore biopsy forceps (1940) (*right*).

over 350 patients." Unfortunately this instrument was considered obsolete within a few years, since both the Schindler esophagoscope and the Eder-Hufford esophagoscope superceded its design.

Given his considerable experience with the design of the gastroscope, Schindler had as early as 1943 sought to improve the esophagoscope. The problem, however, lay in two mutually contradictory design criteria. Firstly the endoscope required a small diameter and a degree of flexibility to assure safety. Secondly, however, if the diameter were limited to 11 mm as with his original 1922 rigid gastroscope, the image provided would be too small to afford adequate visibility. Under these circumstances the logical solution would be to devise a magnifying optical apparatus. After five years of design consultation with ACMI an esophagoscope was produced which conveyed large clear images. It consisted of a rigid hollow tube and obturator with a flexible rubber tip. The finger-like tip facilitated "blind" or palpatory introduction, a procedure already familiar to endoscopists experienced in the use of the Schindler gastroscope. Once the outer tube of the instrument was in place, an inner tube carrying the optical system was inserted. Overall the design was not significantly different to that originally described in 1932 by Norbert Henning. The Henning esophagoscope had, however, met with little acceptance due to a complex but temperamental lens cleaning system. Unfortunately, the Schindler lens system, which was protected by a "clamshell like" cover, also proved to be inadequate and the subsequent modifications which utilized a telescope optical system were introduced too late to forestall the wide acceptance of the Eder-Hufford esophagoscope.

Ray Hufford had begun studying optical systems and obturators for use in rigid esophagoscopes as early as 1943. Within three years he developed a prototype esophagoscope in collaboration with Louis Streifeneder of the Eder Instrument Company. By 1949 adequate preliminary clinical trials and technical refinements had been completed and the Eder-Hufford esophagoscope was introduced. Although it shared many of the features of the Boros and Schindler instruments it was a more serviceable and functional device. It consisted of a rigid outer endoscopic tube and an obturator that ended in a flexible metal coil tipped with a rubber finger. Since this esophagoscope could be introduced in a fashion almost identical to the Schindler semi-flexible gastroscope, American gastroscopists already familiar with the latter device were rapid to accept the Eder-Hufford esophagoscope. A subsequent modification that greatly improved its utility was the introduction of a telescopic optical system (eyepiece) that amplified magnification four-fold and eliminated the problems associated with a lens tube optical system.

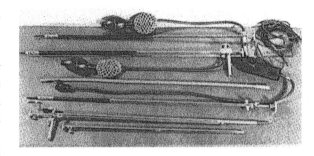

A table set for integrative esophago-gastroscopy (c.1954). The instruments are arranged as follows (*top to bottom*). Eder light-weight flexible gastroscope, Eder Chamberlin Model # 400, drainage tube, Eder-Flexirigid gastroscope, Eder –Hufford flexible esophagoscope with obturator and telescope. In the foreground is a lens obturator and on the right are the rheostat and cords. (*Source: Integrative Esophagogastroscopy, A.R. Hufford Am.J.Gastro.22.1954*)

As a result of the development of a useful instrument for esophageal visualization, the concept of combining the examination of the esophagus and the stomach gained acceptance. Initially it was proposed that both endoscopic procedures might be undertaken with the same instrument or alternatively one instrument might be used for introduction (the esophagoscope) and thereafter the second, the gastroscope, might be passed through it into the stomach. Thus in the early 1950s Eddy Palmer collaborated with Louis Streifeneder in devising the first practical instrument capable of undertaking this dual procedure. Their work culminated in 1953 with the introduction of the Eder-Palmer Trans Esophagoscopic Flexible Gastroscope produced by the Eder Company.

Streifeneder designed two instruments for this purpose, a semi-flexible trans esophagoscopic gastroscope and a rigid trans esophagoscopic gastroscope. Hufford threw his weight behind this concept and within a year had coined the term "integrative esophagogastroscopy." He proposed that the best combination of instruments for this technique would be the Eder-Chamberlin model #400 controlled tip semi-flexible gastroscope used in combination with the Eder-Hufford esophagoscope. Hufford was however broad minded enough to comment that different instruments would probably be adequate depending upon skill and expertise as well as the particular clinical situation. He emphasized that it was "…the responsibility of the esophagogastroscopist to have the training experience and possession of the essential equipment which will enable him to make a complete inspection of the entire esophagus and stomach."

Biopsy or Operating Gastroscope

As early as 1940 Bruce Kenamore had devised a biopsy forceps, which he had successfully used in combination with the Schindler semi-flexible gastroscope. These forceps were not actually a true component of the gastroscope, but were clamped onto the shaft of the endoscope and utilized in conjunction with it. As might be predicted from the "piggy-back" nature of the arrangement, the instrument was subject to mechanical problems and failure. Nevertheless the utility of gastric biopsy to confirm the visual pathology identified either by radiology or gastroscopy was recognized to be an important necessity. In 1948 Edward B. Benedict developed the operating gastroscope which overcame the Kenamore problem by incorporating both a biopsy forceps and a suction tube within the housing of the gastroscope itself.

Modifications were undertaken by I. J. Wood of Australia and by J. Tomenius, who each used a suction tube alone to obtain a mucosal biopsy. Although the addition of the extra channels necessary for the suction and biopsy in Benedict's operat-

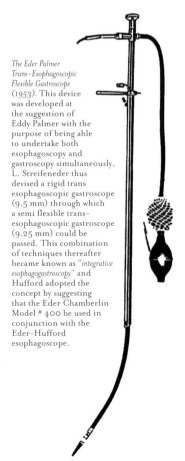

The Eder Palmer Trans-Esophagoscopic Flexible Gastroscope (1953). This device was developed at the suggestion of Eddy Palmer with the purpose of being able to undertake both esophagoscopy and gastroscopy simultaneously. L. Streifeneder thus devised a rigid trans esophagoscopic gastroscope (9.5 mm) through which a semi flexible trans-esophagoscopic gastroscope (9.25 mm) could be passed. This combination of techniques thereafter became known as "*integrative esophagogastroscopy*" and Hufford adopted the concept by suggesting that the Eder Chamberlin Model # 400 be used in conjunction with the Eder-Hufford esophagoscope.

A variety of biopsy forceps. In 1940 Bruce Kenamore had devised a biopsy forceps (*top right*) clamped onto the shaft of the Schindler semi-flexible gastroscope. As might be predicted from the *"piggy-back"* nature of the arrangement, the instrument was subject to mechanical problems and failure. A wide variety of modifications evolved over the years as better techniques of suction and transfixion of tissue were developed.

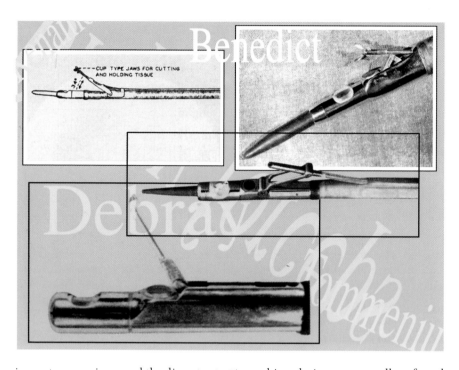

The acquisition of adequate biopsy specimens dramatically decreased the need for exploratory laparotomy as well as removing the need for intellectual guesswork in regard to the pathological nature of radiographic images. As opposed to a determination based on appearance (*top*), advances in staining techniques further amplified the diagnostic yield of biopsy specimens. The acquisition of tissue thus became a vital component of endoscopic technique.

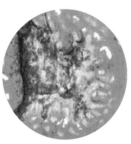

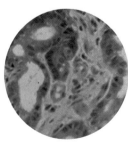

ing gastroscope increased the diameter to 14mm, his technique was overall preferred to that of Wood and Tomenius and remained in use until the early 1960s. Thus Charles DeBrey and Pierre Housset in the *Bulletin of Gastroscopy and Esophagoscopy* (1961) noted that "the instrument most largely used in the United States of America and in the majority of European countries to obtain these delicate mucosal specimens is the Benedict operating gastroscope." Nevertheless, Benedict's device was criticized since its large diameter and oval cross sectional design rendered it difficult to use and uncomfortable for patients. Thus opponents of the operating gastroscope complained that because of its large size and banana shape, it required added technical skill for the physician and increased patient discomfort. Benedict vehemently defended his instrument by claiming that the advantage it offered by generating diagnostic certainty more than justified any of the putative shortcomings.

In addition to the argument regarding the utility of the device, controversy also existed as to whether biopsies were even indicated. Opinions ranged from individuals who believed that biopsy was mandatory in all gastroscopic examinations to those who felt its application was of limited advantage. Benedict himself believed that while gastroscopy should not be regarded as a routine diagnostic procedure, if a gastroscopic examination were to be performed it could not be regarded as complete unless the gastroscopist had some means of biopsy readily available. At the time of Benedict's comments, gastric biopsy was predominantly used to differentiate among gastritis, diffuse carcinoma and lymphoma. The former pathological diagnosis was of considerable importance since prior to the advent of gastroscopy there was no other reasonable method for arriving at this diagnosis and inexplicable symptomatology was the order of the day. Unfortunately, the acquisition of mucosal biopsy material created as much disagreement in regard to the subject of gastritis as the lack of biopsy material. Pathological analysis of inflamed gastric mucosa created pathological controversy and both endoscopists and pathologists struggled (then as now) to establish criteria by which the disease could be recognized.

Irrespective of the tense debate regarding the acquisition of the mucosal biopsy or its pathological interpretation, it was apparent to all gastroscopists that an important diagnostic tool was at their disposal. While biopsy limitations existed, it was evident that considerable potential for information was now available and although biopsy was not accepted as a routine part of gastroscopic protocol, it certainly became more popular. The subsequent advent of both gastroscopic brush cytology and fiber optic instrumentation considerably amplified the application of this important diagnostic technique. Indeed with the increasing sophistication of histologic techniques including immunocytochemistry and electron microscopy, biopsy has become a vital component of the endoscopic process.

ENDOSCOPIC PHOTOGRAPHY

At its inception the development of endoscopic photography revolved around a decision as to whether a camera might be best placed within the stomach or at the external eyepiece. The initial limitations in obtaining photographic documentation reflected shortfalls of the science and technology of photography itself. In 1898 Lange and Meltzung were the first to introduce a small camera into the stomach but the pictures they obtained were of poor quality. Indeed color photography of an acceptable quality within the stomach would only be available some 40 years later in 1937. Prior to this time experimental photography had been possible, but its relative lack of sophistication had precluded successful clinical application. Thus, although many attempts were undertaken during the 1920s, the marginal quality of the image was such that it provided information that was of little diagnostic value. In 1937 Henning and Keilhack produced images of acceptable quality, but in general the overall technique as well as their methodology met with little acceptance. However, in 1948, Harry L. Segal and James S. Watson of the University of Rochester were successful in the construction of an apparatus for the acquisition of color transparencies through a semi-flexible gastroscope.

Their excellent contributions in this area benefited from a substantial collaboration with the local Eastman Kodak Company as well as the Carl Zeiss Company and the Bausch and Lomb Optical Company. These groups provided vital technological support necessary to the development of a functional system. Their contributions included the improvement of the light transmission capability of the gastroscope optics as well as enhancing the light power supply and developing a synchronizing unit in order that changes in the light supply, gastroscope prism, and camera shutter movements could be synchronized. In 1948 Segal and Watson reported in *Gastroenterology* that 61% of the exposures they had taken yielded good color reproduction. This form of technology was further refined over a period of years as photographic devices evolved and miniaturization of components yielded even more useful devices. It remained an acceptable, albeit a somewhat cumbersome mode of obtaining photographic reproduction of the mucosa until the advent of fiber optic technology.

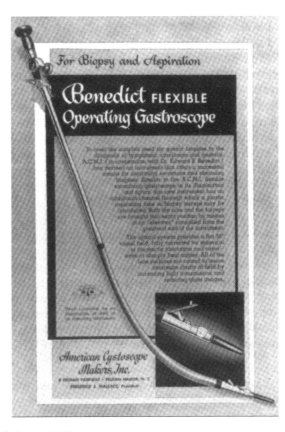

In 1948 E B. Benedict developed the operating gastroscope. A major advantage of this instrument was that it obviated the need for a *piggy back* biopsy device by incorporating both a biopsy forceps and a suction tube within the housing of the gastroscope itself. Critics of the instrument claimed that the addition of the extra channels necessary for the suction and biopsy not only increased the diameter to 14 mm, but also generated a somewhat unwieldy shape and posed a disadvantage. Benedict vehemently defended his instrument by claiming that the advantage it offered by generating diagnostic certainty more than justified any of the putative shortcomings.

The need to preserve the image of the pathology that was viewed was recognized as early as 1898, when Lange and Meltzung attempted to introduce a small camera into the stomach. By the turn of the century, although the Elsner gastroscope had been effectively used for photography, the images were not adequate. Henning and Keilhack in 1937 produced a more effective device for obtaining pictures of the mucosa but the quality was inconsistent and failed to gain acceptance. In 1948 Harry Segal (*background*) and James Watson of Rochester produced a viable endoscopic photographic system (*center*) that could be attached to the eyepiece of the endoscope. This endeavor was undertaken in collaboration with the Eastman Kodak Co., Carl Zeiss Co. and the Bausch and Lomb optical Co. since complex adjustments to lenses, shutters and film were required to adequately capture imagery in the challenging conditions of the gastric lumen.

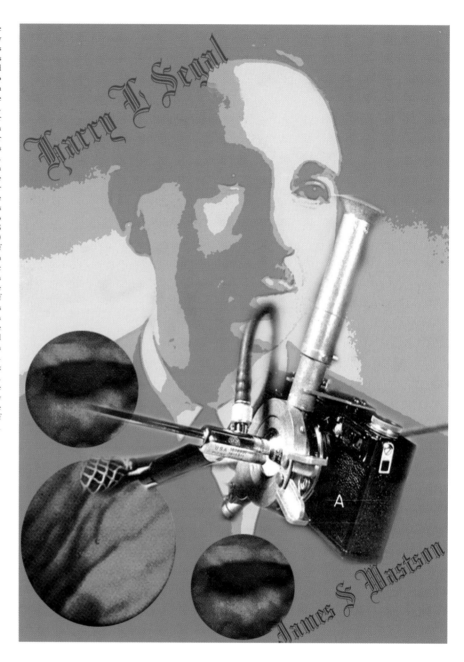

A seemingly exciting further development in this field was presented in 1958 at the first World Congress of Gastroenterology in Washington, D.C. Although the gastro camera had been developed in Japan during the 1950s its debut in the United States was in a large measure due to the enthusiasm of John F. Morrissey, who became a major proponent of this device.

Despite its advanced design and most effective image acquisition, the internal gastro camera device possessed some flaws. Thus, although it yielded excellent photographic images, the endoscopist could neither directly view what was being photographed nor could he be certain that he had acquired the appropriate images until sometime later when the film had been developed. To obviate the former problem the Olympus Corporation in 1963 produced a gastroscope model that featured both fiber optics and a gastro camera within one instrument. Nevertheless the second problem relating to the need for a real time confirmation of adequate documentation still remained unresolved.

The entire issue became moot with the introduction of fiber optic instruments that rendered the gastro camera outmoded since it was apparent that the attachment of an appropriately adapted camera to the endoscope eyepiece could produce direct vision pictures of a quality as high as that of a gastro camera itself. The subsequent advent of video endoscopy rendered both the eyepiece camera and the gastro camera obsolete and provided instantaneous documentation of mucosal conditions.

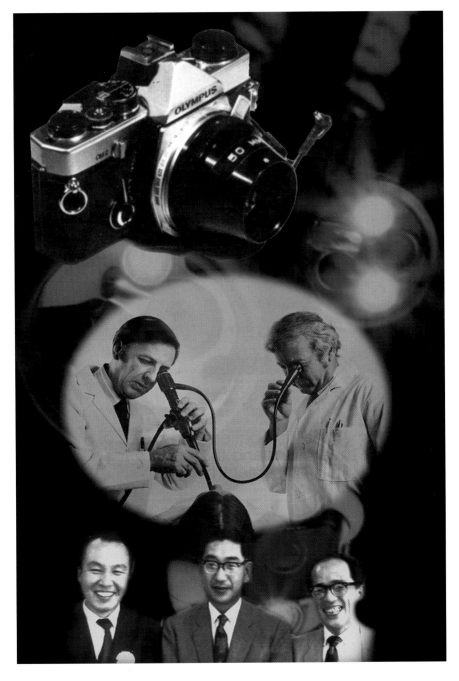

Whereas endoscopic development in the early part of the 20th century had been devoted to the development of flexibility and vision, it was apparent by the 1950's that preservation of the image or transmission of it was of considerable importance. This reflected clinical needs as well as documentation and educational requirements. Corporations such as Olympus Optical Co. not only became involved in the development of endoscopic instrumentation, but also produced cameras specifically designed for endoscopic usage. A particularly innovative concept was the miniature gastrocamera (1952) designed by Tatsuno Uji (*bottom center*) of Japan and his engineering colleagues M. Fukami (*left*) and M. Sugiura (*right*), that could be introduced into the stomach. Despite the brilliance of the concept and the skill of the optical engineering, the disadvantage of the gastrocamera lay in the fact that the user could not see what he was photographing and as result external cameras (*top*) that attached to the eyepiece were developed. By the late 1960's fiber optic technology, umbilical tubes and video endoscopy (*center*) had rendered the use of cameras for the most part redundant.

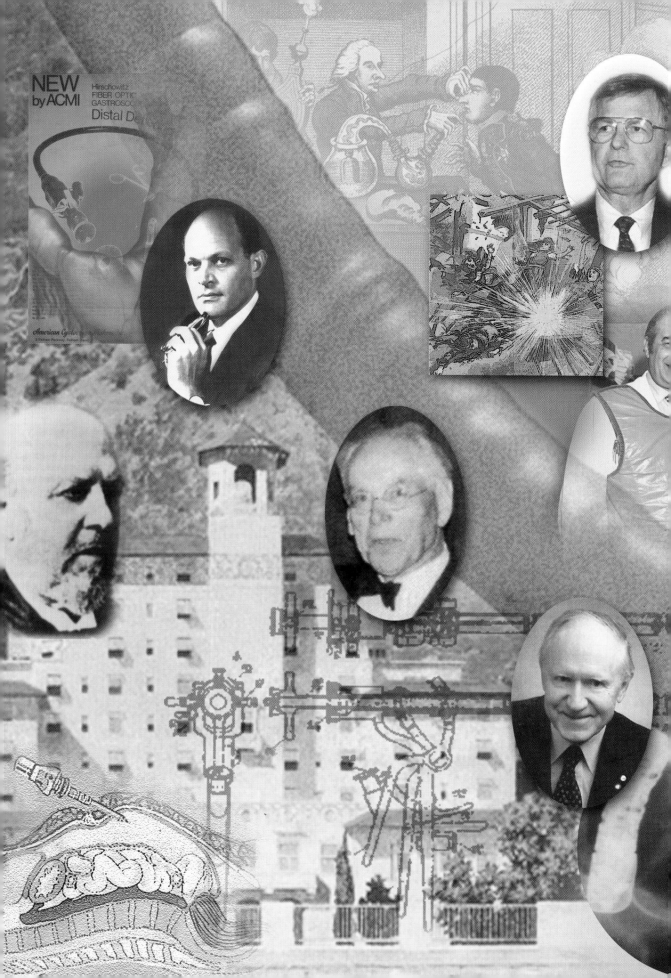

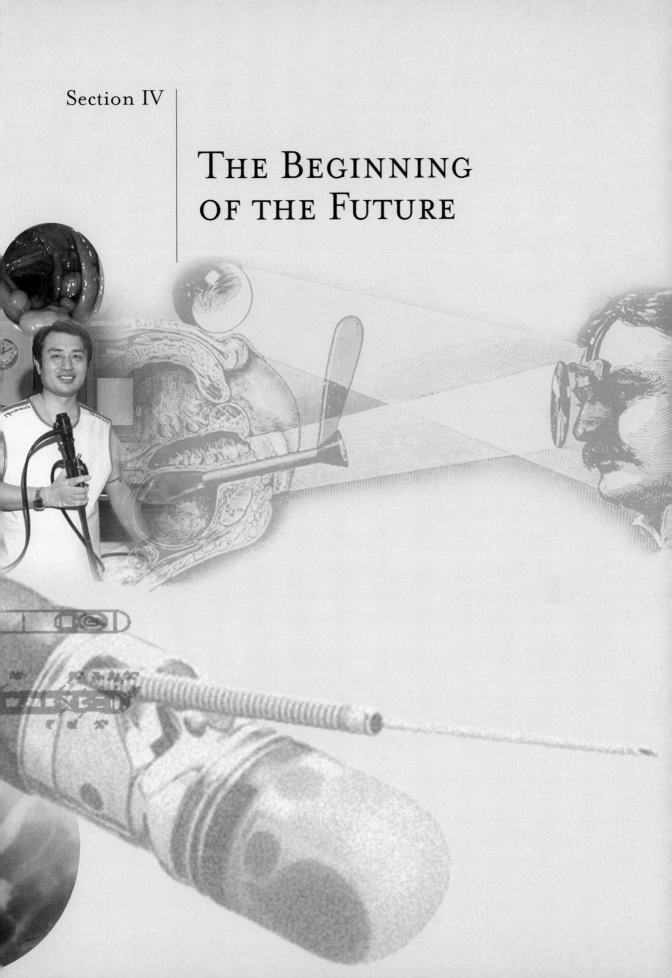

Section IV

THE BEGINNING OF THE FUTURE

CHAPTER I | *Hirschowitz and Fiber Optics*

IN FEBRUARY OF 1957 Basil Hirschowitz passed the first prototype instrument into his own stomach and ushered in the dawn of a new era. After a peripatetic training that began at the University of the Witwatersrand in South Africa, Hirchowitz had obtained specialist skills in the United Kingdom before moving to the United States.

His endeavors in the area of fiber optic endoscopy began in 1954 during a fellowship with Marvin Pollard at the University of Michigan. Having become aware of recent work by Hopkins and Kapany of the Imperial College, London, that dealt with advances in fiber optics, Hirschowitz visited them with a view to discussing the potential applications of fiber optics to endoscopy. Convinced of the feasibility of this concept, Hirschowitz spent the next three years in Ann Arbor working with a physicist, C. Wilbur Peters, and his student, Larry Curtiss, designing and perfecting glass fibers. Thus by 1956 Curtiss had succeeded in producing glass-coated fiber with optical qualities adequate for gastroscope fiber bundle and the construction of a workable model had become feasible. The significant contribution by Larry Curtiss in regard to defining a method by which individual fibers could be optically insulated to facilitate the development of a light transmitting bundle also achieved prominence in the circles of physicists and gastroenterologists alike. Indeed the contributions of Curtiss might be viewed much in the same light as the contributions of Leiter to Nitze's cystoscope or Wolf and Streifeneder's work with Schindler. Schindler himself had previously remarked that arguments as to which were the critical contributions were valueless and that no instrument development could take place without the contributions of either party.

Despite the obvious potential of this application to gastroscopy, the Eder Instrument Company, American Optical and the Genitourinary Manufacturing Ltd. of the United Kingdom declined to become involved. Fortunately in the summer of 1957, ACMI undertook to participate in the initial development of the fiberscope and over the next 3 years design studies were undertaken. By October 1960 the first production model had been developed to a stage considered acceptable for marketing and clinical usage.

Basil Hirschowitz (c. 1957) was born in the Orange Free State, South Africa, obtained a medical degree at the University of the Witwatersrand and trained as a gastroenterologist with Sir Francis Avery Jones in London before assuming a fellowship with Pollard at Ann Arbor, Michigan (*center*), in 1954. As an accomplished gastric physiologist he possessed the intellectual prescience to vault beyond the limitations of a rigid question and perceived the possibilities inherent in the optical work of Hopkins, Kapany and van Heel. Convinced that a fiber optic endoscope could be built, he successfully collaborated with C.W. Peters and L. Curtiss.

This instrument known as the Hirschowitz ACMI 4990 fiberscope was detailed in a 1961 article in the *Lancet* entitled *"The Endoscopic Examination of the Stomach and Duodenal Cap with the Fiberscope"* by Basil I. Hirschowitz. This seminal publication would be the harbinger of a new world of gastroscopy and document the introduction of what would prove to be one of the great contributions of gastroenterology to the world of medicine. Hirschowitz commented within the publication that it was his opinion that "the conventional gastroscope has become obsolete on all counts." Despite nay sayers he was to be proven correct and indeed the veracity of his pronouncement has withstood the ultimate test - time!

Although Hirschowitz had demonstrated his new gastroscope which he called the "fiberscope" at a meeting of the American Gastroscopic Society on May 16th, 1957 at Colorado Springs, the acceptance of the device was not as rapid as might have been predicted. Despite the fact that the President of the Society, John Tilden Howard, actually had the prescience to decline to deliver his Presidential address in lieu of Hirschowitz's historic presentation, the general membership was tardy in its reaction to the innovation. Howard yielded the podium stating: "I shall forego my prerogative of boring you with a presidential address so that Dr. Hirschowitz may at half past 8 o'clock tell you about what I understand to be a new principle of gastroscopy. I hear that fiber glass conducts light around corners and that Dr. Hirschowitz has used this material in a new type of gastroscope". Gastroenterologists in general took a considerable period of time to negotiate this corner themselves.

Initial reports of experience with the fiberscope were guarded in their pronouncements and some even damned it with faint praise. In November 1958 a report comparing the fiberscope and the conventional gastroscope concluded that the former facilitated a better view of the duodenum while the latter afforded a better quality visual image. Robert S. Nelson stated: "it is at present conceded that vision in the duodenum with the fiberscope will probably never be as clear as through the gastroscope in the stomach, but the duodenal ulcer has been reportedly visualized and there is considerable optimism regarding the future development and practical use of the instrument." Even Marvin Pollard who had to some extent participated in Hirschowitz's epic work was somewhat understated in his support of the device. While he accepted that complete flexibility

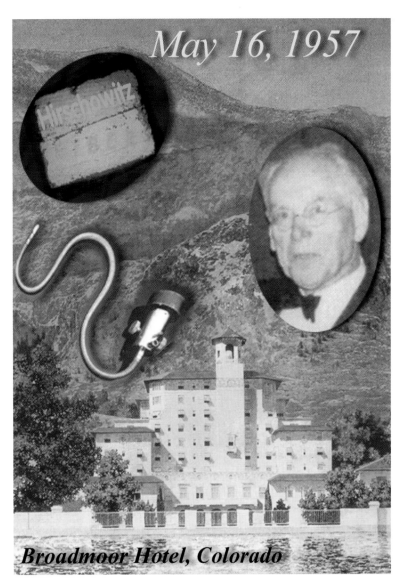

May 16, 1957

Broadmoor Hotel, Colorado

The meeting of the American Gastroscopic Society of May 16th 1957 at the Broadmoor Hotel, Colorado (*background*) was presided over by John Tilden Howard (*right*) and enshrined an epic moment in the history of endoscopy. With a masterful display of humility and prescience Howard yielded the podium and graciously eschewed the privilege of delivering his Presidential Address to enable B. Hirschowitz to present the first demonstration of the *"fiberscope"* to the Society. Due to a major snowfall less than 40 persons witnessed the early morning (8:30 am) presentation of the instrument (*center left*) and a subsequent demonstration of its capability to transmit an image (*top left*). Few present may have realized that they had witnessed the dawn of a new era.

B. Hirchowitz endoscoping a patient (c.1961). In 1959 Hirschowitz moved to Birmingham, Alabama, as Director of the Gastroenterology Unit and much as Birmingham, England had flourished under the intellectual influence of the Lunar Society (Priestley, Watt, Galton, Bolton, Darwin etc) so the endoscopic *cognoscenti* flocked to his doors. In an epic Lancet article of 1961 that assessed the utility of the ACMI 4990 (the model T of fiber optic endoscopy) Hirchowitz claimed to the horror of the Schindlerian Luddites and other inflexible conservatives of the establishment that "the conventional gastroscope is obsolete on all counts." He was right!

In early 1957 Frederick J. Wallace, President of ACMI, agreed to support the development of the fiberscope provided Hirchowitz, Peters and Curtiss would act as consultants. In October of 1960 the first ACMI fiberscope was delivered to Birmingham and within a year the *Lancet* publication documenting its utility established ACMI as the leader in the field. Over the next decade a series of technological modifications (e.g. *distal deflection- 1968*) were introduced at a furious pace.

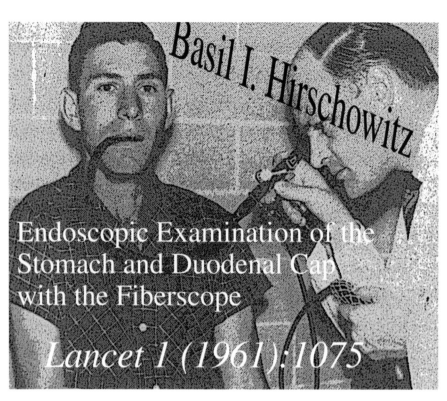

Basil I. Hirschowitz

Endoscopic Examination of the Stomach and Duodenal Cap with the Fiberscope

Lancet 1 (1961):1075

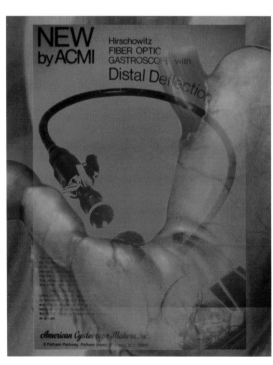

NEW by ACMI Hirschowitz FIBER OPTIC GASTROSCOPE with Distal Deflection

American Gastroscope Makers, Inc.

made it easier for introduction and safer to use and that better light transmission made the photography easier as well as facilitated viewing, he claimed to be uncertain as to whether the duodenum could ever be definitively entered on a predictable basis.

Gastroenterologists were not alone in failing to fully perceive the potential applications of the instrument. John Hett representing the ACMI point of view in 1958 at a meeting of the American Gastroscopic Society stated "...because of the inherent limitation in definition of the fiberscope we believe that its use will be limited to those situations where a conventional optical system is not possible." Contrary to the position of the "nay sayers" comparative studies of the instruments by 1963 had adequately demonstrated that there was little difference in diagnostic accuracy between the two technologies. Despite a substantial body of information supporting the superiority of the fiber optic device, Moses Paulson, in his 1969 textbook of *"Gastroenterologic Medicine"* still demurred and devoted two pages to discussing the comparative benefits and disadvantages of conventional semi-flexible gastroscopes as compared to flexible fiber optic gastroscopes.

Despite Hirschowitz's early optimistic predictions, the ACMI Hirschowitz FO-4990 gastroduodenoscope proved less than ideal in its ability to pass the pylorus into the duodenum. Many who evaluated the device in its early years were in fact quite sanguine in regard to its usage. Norman Cohen and his colleagues reporting in the *American Journal of Digestive Diseases* in 1966 stated that in 1,000 fiberscope examinations that they had been "unable to enter the duodenum with certainty in any examination." Some felt that the endoscope was too big and bulky whilst others complained that it was too flexible. The latter property conferred considerable advantage during introduction but unfortunately provided a tendency to loop in the stomach forming a 'J'. A subsequent model introduced by ACMI (Hirschowitz ACMI 5004 fiberscope) obviated this problem by introducing a controllable tip that was already in place in the semi-flexible conventional models such as the Eder-Chamberlin or Hermon Taylor gastroscope. Indeed the introduction in 1968 of the controllable tip model produced a fiber optic gastroscope that was incontrovertibly more effective in every respect than the previous semi-flexible models.

The decade of the 1970s witnessed a series of rapid technological advances each of which amplified the utility of the endoscope. Although Hirschowitz had first introduced a fiber optic esophagoscope made by ACMI in 1963, Philip A. LoPresti had modified this instrument by 1964 to create the fore-oblique fiber optic esophagoscope. This instrument differed from previous models by altering the angle of vision as well as introducing a channel for suction or instillation of air or water to facilitate insufflating the stomach and keeping the lens clear. Overall the general concept of a forward viewing fiber esophagoscope became transmuted into an endoscope capable of fulfilling all requirements for examination of the upper gastrointestinal tract. In so doing the concept of the panendoscope was finally achieved.

A number of instrument corporations including Olympus Optical Company and Machida joined ACMI in the introduction of a variety of innovative features (length, flexibility, channel size) that added to the utility of the endoscope. By 1971 the length of instruments had been increased to 105 cm (Olympus model GIF) and the duodenum could therefore be routinely visualized. Mobility at the tip was further amplified and the ACMI model 7089P featured a four way control tip and was followed by the 7089J model which increased tip deflection to 180° thus allowing even greater visibility. An especially innovative (but not very popular) concept was the use of a large bore channel through which a small (7 mm) fiberscope could be passed for either diagnostic or surgical procedures. In much the same way as computer technology in the 1990s changed on an almost monthly basis, endoscopy in the 1970s generated technical advances at such a pace that gastroenterologists were barely able to stay abreast of the new possibilities.

Once the fiber optic endoscope was established as a clinical reality, numerous design modifications were added as skillful practitioners of gastroscopy collaborated with instrument makers in amplifying the utility of the device. Thus in 1964 Philip LoPresti of New York (*top right*) modified the Hirchowitz ACMI esophagoscope that had been introduced the previous year introducing a foroblique viewing system as well as a channel for suction and air or water insufflation.

Clinical Experience with a New Foroblique Fiber Optic Esophagoscope

PHILIP A. LoPRESTI, M.D., and AKRAM M. HILMI, M.D.

THE FIBERGASTROSCOPE was the first me... employing the principle of fiber optic... anticipated that other endoscopic instru... utilize the striking flexibility and better lig... system. In conjunction with a manufactu... department has developed a new foroblid... paper will describe the instrument and our... the study of 106 patients (150 examinations)...

THE INSTRUMENT

The instrument is 90 cm. long and 1.1 cm. in dia... are two fiber optic bundles which run the length of the instrument: 3 mm. in diameter, transmits light from an external source to the distal field, and the other, ... as reflected light to the viewing ... ing lens complex (an achromatic objective) is focused by means of a proximal lever. Adjustment of the e... wing lens) may be made to correct for variation in the ob-s... acuity. The external light source is of high intensity and c... by a rheostat control (Fig. 1). Because of the external light s... is no emission of heat at the end of the instrument, and dr... retions on the distal lens (Fig. 2) is not a problem.

CHAPTER 2 | *Video Endoscopy*

98

Early Video Endoscopy by M. Sivak, Cleveland Clinic (c.1984). In much the same fashion as fiber optic endoscopy supplanted conventional semi-flexible instruments in the 1960's, the introduction of microelectronics in the 1980's resulted in the demise of the eyepiece and fiber optically engendered image. Charge coupled devices linked electronically to video processors were embraced as part of the computer age and within a decade the original Welch Allyn prototypes had been replaced by sophisticated instruments manufactured by Fujinon and Olympus and the technology could be found in almost every endoscopy clinic. A further transformation was effected by the direct interface of such systems with more sophisticated computers and resulted in image acquisition, report generation, data management and long distance tele medicine applications.

The technical advances in microelectronics that began in the 1960s were within two decades transferred to the field of gastrointestinal endoscopy. The replacement of an electronic sensor or charge coupled device at the tip of the instrument was introduced in 1983 by Welch Allyn Inc. of Skaneateles of New York. The sensor was designed to transmit an image electronically to a video processor that then displayed the image on a television monitor placed in front of the endoscopist. Initial concerns expressed were much the same as those that had been raised when fiber optic technology was introduced as a replacement to the archaic optical lens systems. On this occasion, however, a new generation of gastroenterologists and instrument makers appeared more susceptible to the introduction of novel technology and less resistance was encountered than had been experienced during the introduction of fiber optic devices 30 years previously. Indeed the rapid recognition of the image discriminant sensitivity using microelectronics rendered the advantages of the acquisition of such technology self-evident. The further development of information transfer systems that allowed for instant image acquisition and storage further confirmed its utility.

More recently the widespread recognition that data transfer as well as data acquisition are critical issues in the management of patients has further propelled endoscopy into the state of the art world of biotechnology. The arduous process of handwritten reports was replaced by dictated reports and thereafter data input using a programmed system with optional input. More recent developments include voice recognition systems, instant photographic records and instant reports. The transmission of information internally or by electronic external mail can facilitate the simultaneous and real time review of information regarding a patient by any physicians involved. Telemedicine devices for long distance evaluation of patient examinations are currently under evaluation and will more than likely within the foreseeable future become a part of daily practice. Further distant but certainly more than feasible will be the introduction of robotic controlled instrumentation that is already advanced in development. Such devices although removing the endoscopist from direct proximity to the patient may make procedures more accessible and expedite care delivery.

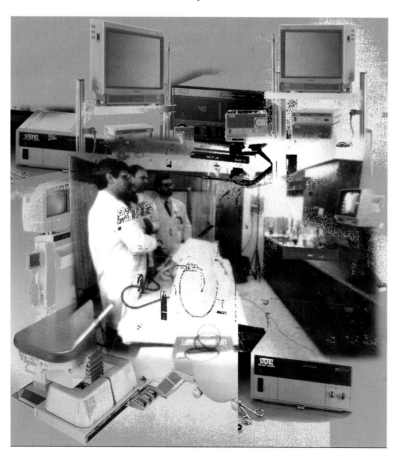

Endoscopic Retrograde Cholangio-pancreatography | Chapter 3

A<small>S A RESULT</small> of improved flexibility of instruments and better visibility, novel opportunities for the examination of the gastrointestinal tract presented themselves to physicians. Having learned to pass the pylorus (keeper of the gateway) and enter the duodenum successfully, identification of the papilla of Vater and the orifice of the pancreatic and biliary duct system soon followed. In 1966 W.C. Watson of Glasgow reported in the *Lancet* his observations of the ampulla Vater and concluded that endoscopic examination might be helpful in the diagnosis of biliary and pancreatic disorders. Although he did not discuss his technique, his suggestions were instrumental in the development of an entirely new diagnostic application of endoscopy. With the territory of the esophagus and stomach now acquired, biopsied and photographed, intrepid endoscopists now sought the *terra nova* of the duodenum, and began the exploration of the interior of the pancreas and hepato-biliary system

In 1965 two radiologists, Rabinov and Simon utilizing a fluoroscopically guided catheter reported the successful per oral cannulation of the papilla of Vater, thus rendering pancreatography a non-operative technique. They noted that since the ampulla could not be regularly visualized fluoroscopically even by use of barium, the technique was arduous and required blind probing of the medial duodenal wall. The situation was problematic since the surgical method of pancreatography was dangerous and difficult, requiring not only a laparotomy but also duodenotomy, while the radiological technique was clumsy, blind and time consuming. In contradistinction, endoscopy had obvious potential advantages in terms of direct visualization.

In 1968 William S. McCune of George Washington University reported in the *Annals of Surgery* experience with successful endoscopic cannulation of the ampulla of Vater. McCune had employed considerable ingenuity to attach a cannula housing onto an Eder fiber optic duodenoscope and was thus able to directly visualize the papilla during the cannulation procedure itself. He commented that "the technique is not easy and requires considerable experience", thus presaging the feelings of endoscopists to this very day. Indeed the initial success rates of McCune and his colleagues for cannulation with this makeshift instrument were less than 50%. The realization of the considerable potential of this procedure led to the rapid development of technical modifications to the duodenoscope that greatly simplified the procedure and by 1970 expert endoscopists were able to claim cannulation rates approaching 90%. The Machida (model FDS) and Olympus (model JF and JFB2) allowed for four way tip control and introduced a lever that facilitated the placement of the cannula into the papilla. In these developmental endeavors the contributions of several innovative Japanese gastroenterologists, including Itaru Oi, T. Takemoto, T. Kondo, and Kunio Takagi, considerably supported the instrument makers.

In 1968 William S. McCune (1909-1998) (*top left*), a surgeon of George Washington University, Washington, published his initial observations with endoscopic retrograde cannulation of the ampulla of Vater in the *Annals of Surgery*. In so doing he opened the doors of perception to the pancreatico-biliary system and provided endoscopists with an entirely new diagnostic and therapeutic vista. The modified Eder fiberduodenoscope used was built in Chicago by an individual named Herman under the guidance of Louis Streifeneder. It possessed both forward and side viewing lenses as well as a tract for the cannula and a balloon that brought the duodenal wall into focus when inflated.

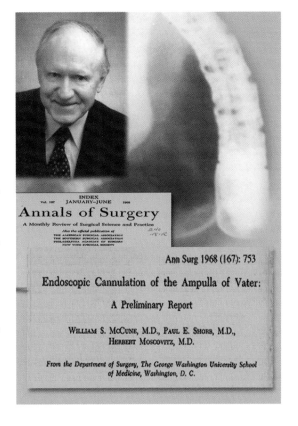

Ann Surg 1968 (167): 753

Endoscopic Cannulation of the Ampulla of Vater:

A Preliminary Report

WILLIAM S. McCUNE, M.D., PAUL E. SHORB, M.D.,
HERBERT MOSCOVITZ, M.D.

From the Department of Surgery, The George Washington University School of Medicine, Washington, D. C.

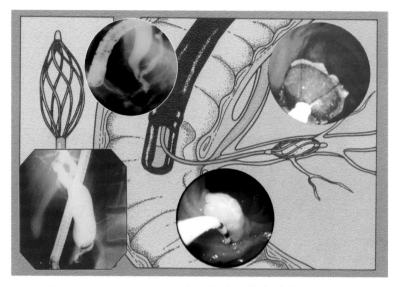

Once the papilla could reliably be cannulated for diagnostic purposes a wide variety of devices were implemented to broaden the therapeutic horizon. The sphincters of Oddi and Boyden were breached by papillotomes; balloons, baskets, stents and coils as a new generation of endoscopists and instrument makers colluded to transluminally supplant the hepato-biliary surgeon. Few would remember the work of the urologist Joaquin Albarran, who in Paris in 1897 had mastered the ureter with almost precisely the same strategies!

Peter Cotton (c. 1985), originally of London and now Charleston, South Carolina, was an early pioneer in the development of ERCP. His maieutic skills and technical innovations led to the widespread application of the technique.

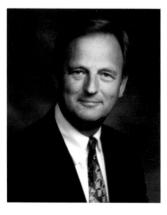

Thus, by 1972, Jack Vennes and Steven E. Silvis were able to publish information pertaining to their first 80 attempts at cannulation and the procedure entered the domain of acceptability in the United States. In 1978 Vennes received the Schindler award from the ASGE in recognition of his contributions to this important new development in gastrointestinal endoscopy.

L. Demling and M. Classen initially conceived the concept of a therapeutic application in 1973, recognizing the major barrier that an intact papilla of Vater constituted for the introduction of therapeutic devices. To split the papilla they developed a high frequency diathermy snare that subsequently became known as the Demling-Classen probe. The device consisted of a Teflon catheter that contained a thin steel wire, which could be protruded to allow for the development of a "bowstring" that served as a diathermy knife. An additional advantage of this probe was the ability to instill contrast medium at the time of the papillotomy and therefore ensure appropriate positioning. Initial canine experiments indicated efficacy and demonstrated that with correct technique a safe papillotomy could be undertaken without bleeding or perforation. Although considerations of scarring were worrisome, further study demonstrated that such events did not occur. At almost the same time K. Kawai of Japan (1973) described a papillotomy device consisting of two diathermy blades of 2-mm length at the tip. This method was particular useful in instances where the stone was impacted in the ampulla itself. In 1974 S. Sohma reported a papillotomy device not significantly dissimilar to that first described by Classen and Demling. This device consisted of a wire, which was not "pulled" to produce a cutting surface but rather "pushed" beyond the tip of the probe. The steel wire therefore ran to the outside of the papillotomy device and when lifted away formed a loop that with appropriate positioning could cut the papillary roof. The Sohma probe became widely used in Japan, but the Erlangen probe remained more popular in the West since it was believed to be safer and less liable to engender perforation.

Although ERCP became widely recognized as an important diagnostic modality, it was apparent that the procedure could be associated with potentially serious complications. A survey conducted in 1974 by the ASGE revealed that the complication rate was at least 2.2% and therefore significantly higher than for any other currently practiced endoscopic technique. Since post ERCP problems included serious events such as pancreatitis, cholangitis, instrument injuries and sepsis, recommendations were provided in an attempt to decrease these complications. Despite the criticisms of those who noted the unacceptably high complication rate, the utility of the procedure in diagnosing pancreatic and hepato-biliary disease provided strong support for its further usage. With the subsequent advent of appropriate training courses and the development of guidelines as well as added experience the complication rate decreased to within acceptable limits.

As endoscopists became more familiar and comfortable with the technique of ERCP as a diagnostic tool, the possibility of therapeutic intervention became a reality. The earliest procedure introduced was that of endoscopic papillotomy using electrocoagulation. Subsequently the removal of biliary calculi was undertaken and a wide variety of techniques and instruments introduced to facilitate this process. All the procedures to extract stones from the common bile duct initially used by surgeons were therefore adapted by endoscopists and instrument makers. By the addition of both flexibility and miniaturization the various devices were modified for introduction through the endoscope channel into the papilla and the need for laparotomy and open choledochotomy obviated. Balloon tipped catheters, back flushing catheters, basket forceps, basket catheters, stone grasping forceps and finally endoscopic laser or ultrasound disintegrators soon became available. The 1975 report by David Zimmon and his colleagues in the *New England Journal of Medicine* describing successful stone removal after endoscopic papillotomy would thereafter open an entire new field of therapeutic endeavor for endoscopists. Indeed as Benedict's operating gastroscope had removed an entire province of surgical endeavor, so would endoscopic papillotomy and biliary exploration ablate yet another significant component of the gastrointestinal surgical armamentarium.

While the development of more sophisticated technique such as CT scan, MRI, isotopic imaging and PET scan have to a certain extent decreased the utility of ERCP as a diagnostic tool, the technique has more than maintained its efficacy by amplification of its therapeutic possibilities. In particular the introduction of biliary and pancreatic stents to either dilate strictures or seal leaks has proved of particular benefit in recent times. Further advances in the use of chemical dissolution and mechanical, electrohydraulic or pulsed dye laser lithotripsy have facilitated the successful management of even the largest and most intractable of biliary calculi. In addition the design and placement of catheters impregnated with high-energy isotopes (Yttrium 90) has raised the issue of even more novel therapeutic possibilities. The likelihood of combined procedures involving both percutaneously introduced steerable catheters by interventional radiologists used in conjunction with transphincterically passed forceps to grasp and manipulate such tubes may result in the development of intraluminal biliary or hepatic surgery in the future.

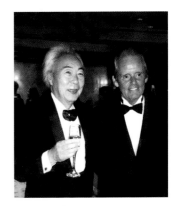

K. Kawai (*left*) of Japan and M. Classen (*right*) of Germany at the 25th Anniversary meeting (Kohler, Wisconsin, 1968) to celebrate the introduction of papillotomy. Their independent successful development of the concept of the technique and instrumentation in 1973 was responsible for an extraordinary advance in biliary and pancreatic therapeutic intervention.

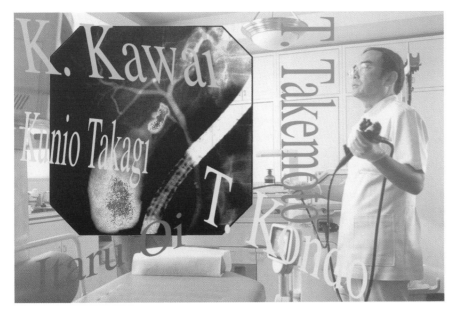

The early experience and innovative development of ERCP and papillotomy by a number of Japanese endoscopists played a prominent role in the worldwide implementation of the techniques. In particular K. Kawai, T. Takemoto, I. Oi, T. Kondo and K. Takagi were preeminent in advancing the field.

CHAPTER 4 | *Colonoscopy*

In 1895 H. Kelly, Professor of Gynecology and Obstetrics at Johns Hopkins University, published in the *Annals of Surgery* the description and drawings of his instruments for procto-sigmoidoscopy. Kelly claimed that the knee-chest position allowed the use of lamplight using a head mirror. The long sigmoidoscope (*center*) permitted ingress to 30 cms and visibility could be improved using the "fecal scooper" (*center vertical*) or the cotton tipped applicator (*left vertical*) to remove mucus. A graded conical sphincter dilator (*top left*) was useful for stricture management and by notation of the gradations therapeutic progress could be assessed.

Instruments to examine the anus and the rectum have been available since the time of the Egyptians and the Romans. Indeed in ancient Egypt the anus was believed to be one of the primary centers of the body wherein health resided. The title "Shepherd of the Anus" was one of the most important positions afforded to physicians of the Royal court of the Pharaohs.

The ruins of Pompeii and Herculaneum have afforded numerous specula whose designs differ little from the modern counterparts of the 19th and 20th centuries. The problems noted in examining the nether regions of the gastrointestinal tract were similar to those encountered in the evaluation of the upper areas. Namely visibility was poor using only reflected lights or candles and in addition the sharp turn of the rectosigmoid junction was a problem not dissimilar to that encountered by the early gastroscopists at the esophagogastric junction and the cricopharyngeal sphincter.

In the United States Howard A. Kelly of John Hopkins University in 1894 introduced the first long (30cm) rigid rectosigmoidoscopes that subsequently became known as "Kelly tubes" by his colleagues. These early devices utilized light from an ordinary oil lamp reflected off a head mirror down the tubular body of the sigmoidoscope.

In 1903 James P. Tuttle of New York in association with the Electro Surgical Instrument Company of Rochester, developed a rectosigmoidoscope with an integrated electric lighting system. A variety of such devices was subsequently produced and included the Strauss proctosigmoidoscope, manufactured by Georg Wolf of Berlin, as well as the Lynch proctosigmoidoscope made by the Electro Surgical Instrument Company.

While such instruments provided relatively good visibility for diagnostic purposes as far as the rectosigmoid junction, attempts to pass beyond this met with difficulty and often resulted in perforation. Even if the junction were successfully negotiated, access beyond 25-30cm could not be gained due to the limitations imposed by the rigidity of the instrument, the acute angulation of the rectosigmoid junction and the curvature of the sigmoid colon. It had been demon-

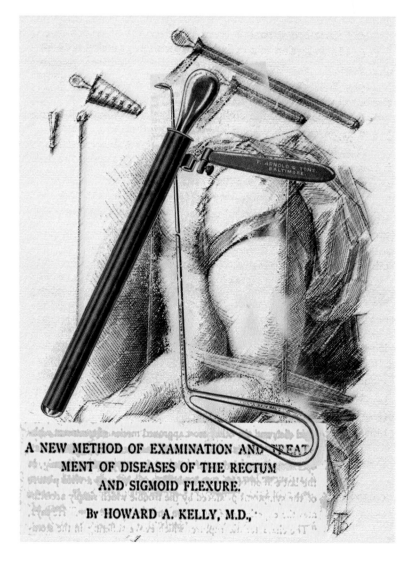

A NEW METHOD OF EXAMINATION AND TREAT-
MENT OF DISEASES OF THE RECTUM
AND SIGMOID FLEXURE.

By HOWARD A. KELLY, M.D.,

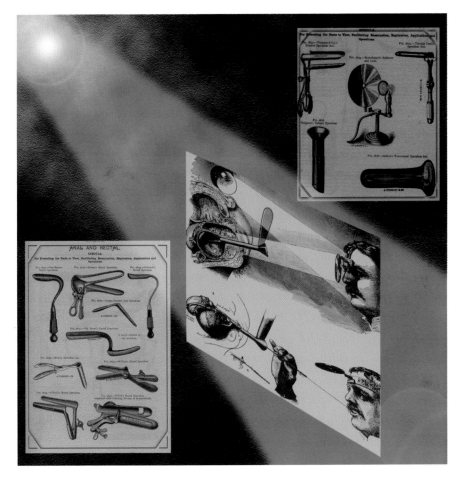

The examination and care of the nether region had been of considerable concern to humans since the distant times of the Egyptians. Thus the Chester Beatty papyrus is devoted solely to ano-rectal disease and the great physician Irj (Ir-en Akhty) of the 10th dynasty is recorded as carrying the illustrious title of "Shepherd of the Anus". Examples of a wide variety of rigid instruments had been developed over the centuries ranging from the hollow wooden pipes of African tribes to the diverse specula of Greece and Rome. Nevertheless, irrespective of material or design, inadequate lighting and flexibility proved critical obstacles to ingress beyond the rectosigmoid junction. In addition the length and tortuosity of the colon further accentuated the limitations of rigid devices prior to the widespread introduction of fiber optic technology in the early 1960's.

strated in 1928 by H.C. Hoff that a flexible tube could be passed as far as the cecum under radiological control. Although this blind procedure was of little diagnostic use to endoscopists, it did indicate that retrograde transmission of a device from anus to cecum was possible. In 1957, F. Matsunaga had attempted to use a modified gastro camera to intubate the colon, but this technique was difficult, provided only modest information, and did not meet with widespread acceptability. The advent of the fiberscope of Hirschowitz in 1957 allowed for the serious consideration of fiber optic sigmoidoscopy and colonoscopy.

By the early 1960s the Machida and Olympus Corporations developed proto-type models which were evaluated in the United States and Japan. Market versions of these devices were introduced in 1965 and a prominent role in their adoption was provided by the contributions of Oshiba, Kanazawa, Niwa and Wantanabe.

Of particular interest in 1965 was a report of the first total colonoscopy per-formed in a human subject by Luciano Provenzale and Antonio Revignas of Cagliari University, Sardinia, Italy. In a highly innovative fashion their subject was induced to swallow a doubled long polyvinyl tubing which over a period of days emerged from his anus. Provenzale and his colleague then attached the tubing via a pulley sling to a side viewing Hirschowitz gastroscope and gently pulled it northwards through the entire colon up to the cecum. Although this succeeded in its goal of achieving total colonoscopy, the technique was generally regarded as unacceptable for routine usage.

Although the island of Sardinia (*left*) had languished in relative obscurity since the departure of the Carthaginians, the innovative contributions in 1966 of Luciano Provenzale and Antonio Revignas (*top left*) of the University of Cagliari to the development of colonoscopy once again reminded the world of the power of the heirs of the Caesars. Using the 1955 technique of Blankenhorn for end to end intestinal intubation, with a small caliber swallowed tube they positioned a pulley system of thin polyvinyl tubing arranged in tandem in the digestive tract and attached it to a lateral viewing, non-steerable Hirschowitz gastroscope. The application of a light pulling or pushing force enabled the gastroscope to progress endolumenally in a retrograde fashion along the length of the colon (*center*).

In 1963 Robert Turell reported his experiences with a fiber optic illumination system in a colonoscope and a sigmoidoscope in the *American Journal of Surgery*. Although the "flexible fiber optic colonoscope" which he described was little more than a Hirschowitz ACMI gastroscope adapted for use as a colonoscope, it nevertheless represented the first application of fiber optics to colonoscopy. Despite his pioneering efforts in this area Turell nevertheless expressed reservations about the application and development of a flexible instrument for colonoscopic use. In 1967 (four years after his initial publication) he reported "at the present time the flexible fiber optic scope is undergoing extensive studies and unlike the rigid sigmoidoscope, is not yet ready for routine clinical use." Fortunately for endoscopy, Bergein F. Overholt was more confident of the future possibilities of this instrument and working in conjunction with the Eder Instrument Co. developed a flexible fiber optic sigmoidoscope whose application he presented at the ASGE meeting in Colorado Springs, Colorado in May 1967. Convinced that better illumination, adequate flexibility and deeper penetration would all be to the advantage of both the endoscopist and the patient, Overholt within two years reported favorably on the newly introduced Olympus colonoscope (model CF-SB).

By 1970 a longer version of this instrument had been introduced that in addition possessed the additional feature of a four-way tip deflection that facilitated negotiation of the colonic flexures. By 1970 investigators in Japan, Britain, and elsewhere in the United States had enthusiastically endorsed Overholt's experience with the Olympus instrument and participated in further modifications of its

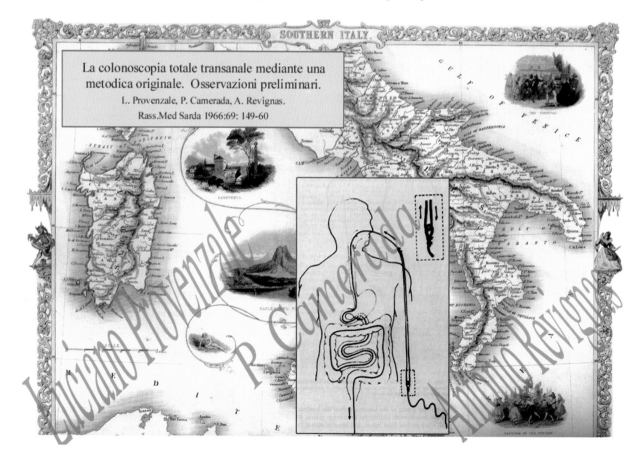

La colonoscopia totale transanale mediante una metodica originale. Osservazioni preliminari.

L. Provenzale, P. Camerada, A. Revignas.

Rass.Med Sarda 1966:69: 149-60

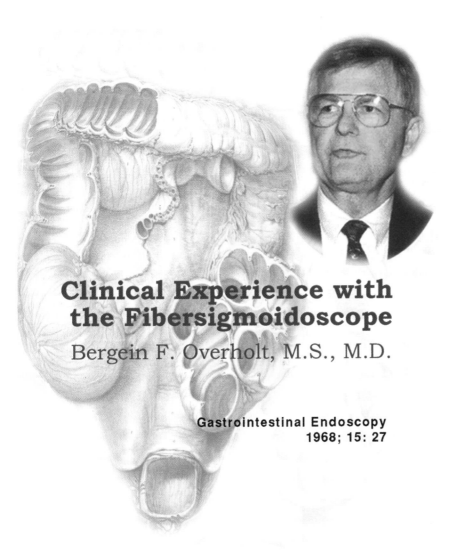

Clinical Experience with the Fibersigmoidoscope

Bergein F. Overholt, M.S., M.D.

**Gastrointestinal Endoscopy
1968; 15: 27**

Although Robert Turell, a surgeon at the Albert Einstein College of Medicine, NYC, had in 1963 used a modified flexible gastroscope to access the left colon, he did not pursue the matter further. Thereafter Susanne Lemire and Arthur E. Cocco of Baltimore (1966) reported their experience with inspection of the left side of the colon using an Eder fiber optic gastroscope for the purpose. Bergein Overholt (*top right*) at the University of Michigan, Ann Arbor, had in 1961 begun to work on the application of fiber optic technology to visualization of the colon. By 1963 he had used the flexible sigmoidoscope clinically and in May of 1967 Overholt presented his initial experience to the American Society for Endoscopy. The published material (*center*) attested to the progress made in the manufacture of the device and confirmed its superiority to rigid sigmoidoscopy. The initial contributions of Overholt would help define colonoscopy as one of the most important diagnostic techniques of the 20th century.

design. George Berci and his colleagues in 1971 as well as William Wolff and Hiromi Shinya reported excellent results that documented not only complete examination of the colon but also an absence of any complications. Further modifications of the short and long colonoscope resulted in modifications of the flexibility as well as the introduction of omni-directional viewing with four-way tip deflection. Some skeptics still proposed a place for the rigid sigmoidoscope, but by the late 1970s almost all endoscopists had concluded that fiber optic sigmoidoscopes or colonoscopes were superior in almost all circumstances. As always issues of training and experience entered into the evaluation of data, but most parties concluded that the diagnostic information yielded by the fiber optic instrument far outweighed any possible difficulties encountered in the initial time required to learn its usage.

Such considerations were further supported by the fact that colon cancer was recognized as the most common form of internal cancer in the United States, with more than a 100,000 new cases being diagnosed annually and 8 to 15% of the adult population possessing colonic polyps. Under the circumstances it seemed both timely and appropriate that the fiber optic colonoscope become the diagnostic tool of choice. In this respect the discussion of the colonoscope as a diagnostic modality had virtually been pre-empted by the innovative therapeutic work of William I Wolff and Hiromi Shinya. In 1971 at the Beth Israel Hospital, New York, they successfully undertook the removal of colonic polyps with a wire loop snare in the biopsy channel of a fiber optic colonoscope.

Within a year they were able to report a further 300 polypectomies with minimal complication rates and zero mortality. The recognition that polyps represented pre-cancerous lesions and that polypectomy might now be safely undertaken in many circumstances without resort to laparotomy or colectomy was regarded as a dramatic advance. Although more cautious individuals initially insisted that colonoscopic polypectomy was being practiced over enthusiastically and that bleeding, perforation and gas explosions were common complications, a detailed analysis of the available data failed to support such conclusions. Indeed Wolff rebutted such statements vehemently in the *New York State Journal of Medicine* of 1973 noting that he had undertaken 1600 polypectomies without complication. His personal experiences were vindicated in a 1974 ASGE survey that revealed that in 6,200 polypectomies there had been no mortality and the overall number of complications were extremely low. No documentation of any colonic gas explosion could be identified and polypectomy was unanimously vindicated as a procedure that had come of age.

CHROMOENDOSCOPY AND MAGNIFICATION ENDOSCOPY

The constant search for better methods to evaluate pathological changes in the mucosa has led to the development of magnification endoscopy and chromoendoscopy. The first magnifying colonoscope was described by Tada in 1975 and had the ability to magnify 10 times. The models developed subsequently have considerably increased magnification capability and when used in combination with various dyes have allowed for the recognition of subtle alterations in mucosal pattern. Dyes which have been utilized include either absorptive stains which enter the cell by diffusional absorption or reactive stains which interact with the epithelium to produce a characteristic color change based upon a chemical reaction (Congo red). A third type, contrast stains, are not absorbed and do not react with the surface mucosa but disperse into mucosal elevations and depressions providing a specific topographic appearance. A variety of dyes including methylene, toluidine blue (stain dysplastic tissue), indigo carmine, which demonstrates the set patterns of the crypt of Lieberkuhn of both the mucosa and polyps have been utilized. The dyes can be either

William Wolff (*right*) and Hiromi Shinya (*left*) (c. 1975) of the Beth Israel Hospital, New York (*background*) were not only instrumental in developing safe and effective colonoscopy, but convincingly demonstrated that polypectomy was not only a feasible procedure but safe and effective. Although the concept of polypectomy was initially criticized, the publication of a series of carefully documented patient studies and reviews (*top left*) led to the widespread acceptance of therapeutic colonoscopy. There is little doubt that their contributions dramatically impacted upon the issues of colon cancer surveillance and prophylaxis.

CURRENT PROBLEMS IN SURGERY

MODERN ENDOSCOPY of the ALIMENTARY TRACT

William I. Wolff
Hiromi Shinya

administered orally with the colonic lavage solution, as in the case of indigo carmine, or else focally sprayed upon an area thought to represent abnormal or dysplastic tissue. The simultaneous use of a magnifying colonoscope with an adjustable focusing system enables a close-up view of a mucosal surface which can be magnified from between 10 to 35 times. Ultra high magnification scopes can increase this to 170 times and thus provide dramatic visual images of the mucosa. A further advance has been the development of high resolution endoscopic instrumentation thus the standard of 100,000 to 200,000 pixels may be amplified to greater than 400,000. Under such circumstances diagnostic accuracy to identify dysplastic lesions has been considerably increased. In addition the ability to differentiate adenomatous (sulcus pattern) from hyperplastic polyps with a characteristic pitted pattern is over 90%. A problem of such high resolution instrumentation, however, is the fact that it is not compatible with all endoscopic systems and not as easy to intubate the cecum.

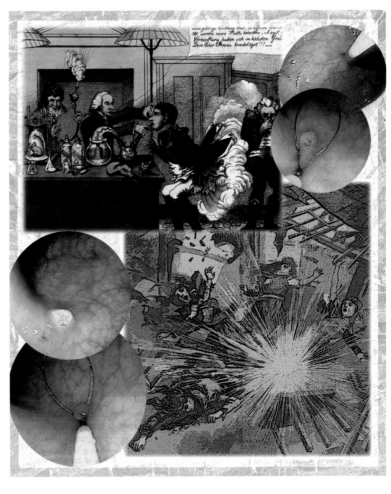

Of particular interest is the use of both methylene blue and indigo carmine to detect and highlight flat adenomas or carcinomata. Given the importance of small flat lesions in the spectrum of colonic neoplasia, the use of chromoendoscopy has been a valuable addition in these areas. The use of indigo carmine dye spread on the mucosal surface in difficult areas such as ulcerative colitis has provided a valuable method to define areas of active histologic change as compared to adjacent areas with healed histologic features. Since the identification of a polyp or an abnormal mucosal area leads to biopsy and histological examination, such techniques are costly. Thus dye spraying and magnification technology may prove valuable screening tools and significantly decrease the cost of colon cancer screening programs.

Polypectomy (*left bottom and right top*) engendered a number of concerns among physicians. Anxiety in regard to perforation and bleeding was rife and prophets of doom (boom) predicted internal implosion due to inflammable colonic gas. The early experiments of R. Lavoisier with explosive gas no doubt fueled such speculation [*top left*: Satirical 19th century, German cartoon depicting Lavoisier experimenting on Napoleon (*right*)]. Such concerns were soon dispelled and for the most part represented long standing societal concerns (mostly of Freudian origin) regarding scybala and flatus.

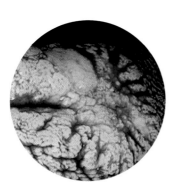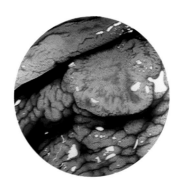

The use of dye sprays including toluidine and methylene blue together with magnification has facilitated the demonstration of the mucosal architectural pattern. Such techniques have greatly increased the ability to detect dysplasia, determine the nature of polyps and define flat carcinomatous lesions.

CHAPTER 5 | *Laparoscopy*

DIMITRI OSKAROVICH OTT, who used a gynecological head mirror and speculum to perform the procedure, undertook the first documented laparoscopy in 1901 in Petrograd. Ott termed the procedure a "ventroscopy" and others have subsequently used terms including peritoneoscopy, celioscopy, and organoscopy. George Kelling of Dresden, who was active both in esophagoscopy and gastroscopy, is regarded as the first to introduce this technique as a gastrointestinal diagnostic procedure. In 1902 he reported examining the peritoneal cavity of a dog using the Nitze cystoscope but by 1910 had undertaken a number of successful laparoscopies on patients. Kelling's contributions were substantial in that he described the methodology for safely inducing a pneumoperitoneum as well as the location and appropriate methodology of port placement. Subsequently in 1910 Hans Christen Jacobaeus coined the term "laparoscopy", which supplanted the previously utilized term "Koelioskopie" that had been utilized by Kelling. Jacobaeus was enthusiastic about the utility of the procedure and in his experience with 45 patients reported the successful diagnosis of cirrhosis, tuberculosis peritonitis, metastatic tumors and even Pick's disease. One year later in 1911 at the John Hopkins Hospital, Bertram Bernheim undertook the procedure that he chose to refer to as "organoscopy". Bernheim, like his predecessors, was limited by the fact that the instrument he utilized was a cystoscope with a limited angle of vision of 90°.

In 1912 S. Nordentoeft of Copenhagen designed an instrument which he called a trocar endoscope. In principle the method was identical to that of G. Kelling, H. C. Jacobaeus and B. Bernheim, but use of the Trendelenburg position improved visibility allowing inspection of the depths of the female pelvis. F. Tedesko presented further

Although Dimitri Oskarovich Ott, a gynecologist of St Petersburg, Russia, is credited with undertaking the first laparoscopy (he called it ventroscopy) in 1901, it was George Kelling of Dresden, Germany (*top right*) who most effectively demonstrated its clinical applicability. In 1901 at the *73rd German Naturalists and Physicians* meeting Kelling demonstrated its usage on a live dog by inserting a Nitze cystoscope into the peritoneal cavity and demonstrating the pristine condition of the abdominal viscera. Although Kelling referred to his technique as "*coelioscopy*" in his January 1902 publication (*top left*), it would subsequently be variously recognized as organoscopy or peritoneoscopy. By 1910 Kelling had devised a safe technique for inducing pneumoperitoneum, produced modified instruments (*bottom*) and successfully examined a series of humans.

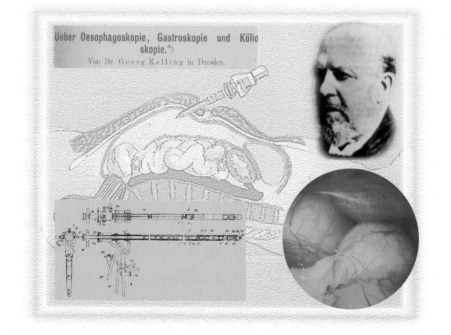

Ueber Oesophagoskopie, Gastroskopie und Kölioskopie.*)
Von Dr. Georg Kelling in Dresden.

information on the subject of laparoscopy in 1912 at the Society of Internal Medicine and Pediatrics in Vienna, but the audience for the most part rejected the procedure as dangerous. In 1913 L. Renon and G. Rosenthal of France published papers of both thoracoscopy and laparoscopy. Their preoccupation however was more with the former and Renon in fact believed that while laparoscopy was useful for visualizing the liver, he doubted whether it would be of use in other intraperitoneal observations. A. Roccavilla of Italy provided a major advance in 1914 by modifying Kelling's methodology and designing an instrument that maintained the light source outside the abdomen. Light was directed down the trocar into the peritoneal cavity by reflection. In 1920 R.H. Orndorf of Chicago published his extensive experience on laparoscopic technique using it in conjunction with a Roentgen screen. His major contribution however was the design of a sharp pyramid point to be used on the trocar.

In 1921 R. Korbsch of Berlin developed novel instruments and technical ideas including a separate pneumoperitoneum needle. Of interest is the fact Korbsch was the first to show colored peritoneoscopy pictures that had been painted by his artist. The following year Unverricht of Germany in publishing his extensive experiences on laparoscopy and thoracoscopy noted that the former would be more acceptable if a wider diameter visual field and stronger light were available. R. Zollikofer of Switzerland in 1924 introduced the use of carbon dioxide for insufflation recognizing that it was absorbed more rapidly. Z.E. Stone of Kansas in 1924, claiming to be unaware of the experiments in Europe, utilized a nasopharyngoscope for laparoscopy and in addition fitted the outer portion of the trocar with a rubber gasket to prevent gas leakage. In the same year O.P. Steiner of Atlanta, Georgia, published a paper entitled "Abdominoscopy" and claimed that he had been unable to identify any other previous publications either theoretical or practical dealing with the subject. Although he indicated that he had discovered an entirely new diagnostic technique, which had never been previously utilized, his work was little different from that of Kelling. In 1925 O.E. Nadeau and O.F. Kampmeier of Chicago published a paper entitled "Endoscopy of the Abdomen" and provided an extensive review of the literature. They noted that although laparoscopy was widely used in Europe "the method was seldom used" in America. In England, A. R. Short in 1925 used a cystoscope to visualize the abnormal organs and felt "the potential of such endoscopic exploration was too fascinating not to explore." Adequate vision however remained a critical problem. Kremer first addressed this limitation in 1927 by modifying the instrument to a forward viewing device and in 1929 Kalk devised an effective new system of lenses which further increased the viewing angle to 135°. His prolific contributions to the field over the next 20 years earned him the sobriquet of "The Father of Laparoscopy."

Despite the unique clinical possibilities that might be provided by the development of this instrument, its design would remain essentially unchanged for the next 30 years, apart from some modifications introduced in the 1930s by John C. Ruddock and Edward B. Benedict, who were enthusiastic supporters of the technique. In 1934 Ruddock initiated a collaboration with ACMI that entailed modification of the McCarthy cystoscope with the

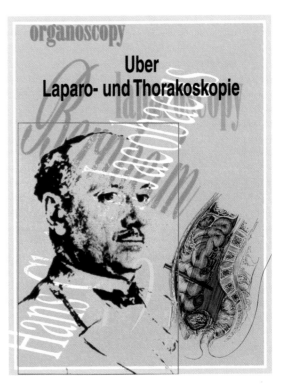

In 1910 Hans Christen Jacobaeus of Stockholm (left) and published 2 cases of visceral exploration; one thoracic and one abdominal and designated his technique as thoraco-laparoscopy ("Über Laparo- und Thorakoskopie"). The methods he used were less advanced than Kelling, who had described a separate needle with filtered air to produce the pneumoperitoneum, preferring to use the trocar for this purpose. Although Jacobaeus reported on 115 laparoscopies in 1912 and described cirrhosis, metastatic disease and tuberculous peritonitis, he thereafter abandoned the procedure and devoted his attention to thorascopic lysis of tuberculous lung lesions. The logic of the latter procedure proposed that lysis would permit complete lung collapse after artificial pneumothorax induction and thereby ensure healing!

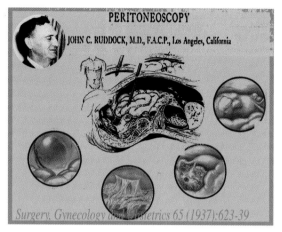

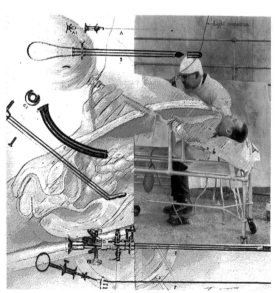

John Ruddock of Los Angeles (*top left*) became a major proponent of laparoscopy, although E. Benedict of Boston published prolifically on the subject. To facilitate peritoneoscopy, as he preferred to call it, Ruddock modified a McCarthy cystoscope, redesigned the trocar and biopsy instruments and used local anesthesia. In 1937 he documented his initial experiences with 500 patients. By the end of his career he had reported more than 2500 cases with excellent results and low complication rates.

O. Nadeau of Chicago (*right*) (c. 1925) undertakes laparoscopy on a patient under local anesthesia. The collage of instruments is representative of the diverse array available for examining the peritoneal cavity and abdominal viscera.

addition of a fore-oblique visual system to facilitate viewing the peritoneal cavity. Ruddock termed his device a "peritoneoscope" and in 1937 published details of 500 cases that he had undertaken. He claimed that usage of the instrument had increased his diagnostic accuracy from 63.9% to 91.7% and in addition and most importantly, had avoided the expensive and dangerous necessity of a laparotomy. Edward Benedict of Boston had already made powerful statements regarding the utility of gastroscopic biopsy for obtaining diagnostic information and took a similar position in support of laparoscopy. He enthusiastically advocated its extensive use in the diagnosis of gastrointestinal disease as well as noting its obvious gynecological applications. Nevertheless the relatively clumsy nature of the instruments as well as the limited visibility of some areas of the peritoneal cavity obviated the widespread acceptance of this technique.

Such considerations were however to a large extent mollified by the advance of technology in the early 1950's. Thus in 1952, when N. Fourestier and his associates introduced the use of a quartz light rod to replace the distal lamp in the bronchoscope, it became apparent that the future was at hand. The application of this novel method of light transmission to diverse endoscopic instruments including laparoscopes provided not only brilliant illumination but obviated the heat problems that had been generated by the distal lamp. Similarly the introduction of the quartz light rod not only amplified illumination but also eliminated electrical hazards and facilitated the use of color cinematography and television imagery in the peritoneal cavity. A draw back of the quartz rod, however, was its high price, fragility and the need to position the light source in close proximity to the external eyepiece. While these issues were under examination the entire matter became moot with the introduction of the fiber optic bundle by Hirschowitz in 1957. The widespread introduction of fiber optic technology to laparoscopy was thereafter combined with the development of flexible tip instruments. In 1981 Robert A. Sanowski and his colleagues modified a pediatric Olympus endoscope for use as a laparoscope and demonstrated that the endoscope was readily adaptable to laparoscopy without major modification. These studies were however superceded by the development of instruments designed specifically for diagnostic and therapeutic application within the peritoneal cavity. In this respect the United States Surgical Company and Ethicon played a substantial role in masterminding a gastrointestinal surgical renaissance by developing novel instruments that facilitated the interface of the disciplines of endoscopy and surgery. Thus laparoscopy moved from a humble and cumbersome diagnostic procedure in the early 1980s to become the state of the art technique for cholycystectomy, fundoplication, splenectomy, colectomy and a wide variety of anastomoses within a decade.

The cycle whereby laparotomy, initially a diagnostic procedure, in the early part of the century was supplanted by endoscopy and laparoscopy has now attained the full circle whereby laparoscopy has become transmogrified from a diagnostic procedure into one with major therapeutic applications. Issues of what training and expertise are required to differentiate those who would undertake diagnostic procedures versus therapeutic are still matters that require resolution.

Percutaneous Endoscopic Gastrostomy | CHAPTER 6

THE EARLIEST PERCUTANEOUS access to the human stomach was provided by either incidental trauma or disease. Thus Jacob Helm of Vienna reported his experience of studying the digestion of Theresa Peitz in 1803 when she presented with a spontaneous gastric fistula. William Beaumont studied Alexis St. Martin in 1822 after the latter had acquired a musket induced gastric fistula and Nicolas Blondlot in 1843 successfully constructed a canine gastrostomy for the formal study of gastric secretion. Although the Russian physiologist W. Bassow was the first to propose the utility of a human gastrostomy, Charles Sédillot in 1849 was the first to successfully undertake the procedure. The operation was thereafter popularized by A. Vernuil (1876) and Charles Richet (1878) and K. Lennander (1908), who respectively demonstrated the efficacy of the procedure to either provide nutrition or drain an obstructed stomach. Over the next three decades gastrostomy became regarded as a popular and useful technique and a wide variety of surgical modifications were developed in the early 20th century to provide long-term access to the stomach. Such operative procedures supplanted the chronic use of stomach tubes and were of particular utility in feeding patients who could not swallow or for the decompression of stomachs obstructed by pyloric pathology. Despite being a relatively modest surgical technique, morbidity and mortality were substantial given the patient population that required such intervention

In 1980 Jeffrey Ponsky and Michael W. L. Gauderer described an "incisionless gastrostomy" that had been developed for long term internal feeding of pediatric patients at the Children's Hospital in Cleveland. Their novel procedure involved a percutaneous needle puncture of the gastric wall, through which a suture was passed into the stomach before being withdrawn by an endoscope out of the patient's mouth. The gastrostomy tube attached to this line was then drawn retrograde down the esophagus through the stomach wall and secured at the puncture site in the abdominal wall. So effective and safe has this procedure become that in 1990 it was estimated to be the second most common indication for upper endoscopy in hospitalized patients in the United States. Indeed the efficacy of the maneuver has been such that surgical gastrostomy has virtually become a technique of the past. Although other methods of percutaneous endoscopic gastrostomy have been described using either radiographically guided introduction or push techniques the principle first introduced by Ponsky has become widely adopted as one of the most significant therapeutic procedures in the armamentarium of the endoscopist.

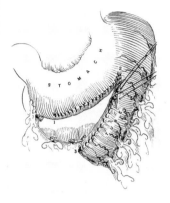

A Beck Jianu Surgical Gastrostomy. For almost a century continual access to the stomach in cases of gastric outlet obstruction or esophageal disease could only be attained by the construction of a gastrostomy. A wide variety of such stomas had been devised (each with its proponents and critics). All however required major surgical intervention and were associated with a substantial morbidity and even mortality.

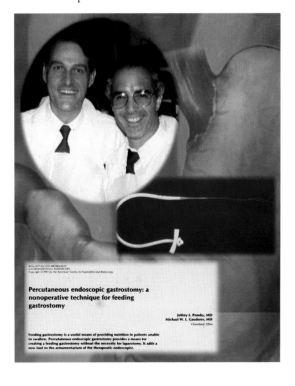

Jeffrey Ponsky, general surgeon and endoscopist (*right*), and Michael Gauderer, pediatric surgeon (*left*), conceived and perfected a novel technique (1980) to obviate the need for open surgical construction of a gastrostomy. Although initially contemplated as a pediatric procedure, it was soon widely adopted in adults as a well tolerated, efficacious and low risk intervention. Standard operative gastrostomy, like peptic ulcer surgery, thereafter faded for the most part from the armamentarium of the general surgeon. The center insert is the original tube used in the first PEG. (*Courtesy J. Ponsky*)

CHAPTER 7 | *Endoscopic Ultrasound (EUS)*

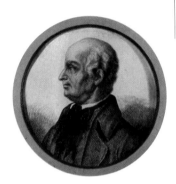

Lazzaro Spallanzani (1729-99). A cleric and polymath he initially studied law at Bologna, before switching to physics, theology and then Natural History. Included in his manifold contributions are the description of the physiological basis of digestion (1780) and the discovery of artificial insemination.

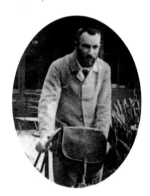

Pierre Curie (1859-1906), Professor of Physics, Sorbonne, Paris was the husband of Marie Curie and joint Nobel prize winner with her and Antoine Becquerel.

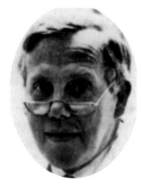

John J. Wild, an Englishman working at the University of Minnesota (1950), was the first to demonstrate the difference between normal and malignant bowel tissue using ultrasound.

In 1794 L. SPALLANZANI noted that bats at night flew without striking obstacles and proposed that their guidance system was auditory rather than visual. Since no sound was evident, he concluded that the sound was beyond human auditory perception! Pierre and Jacques Curie in 1880 discovered the piezoelectric effect, whereby mechanical pressure on quartz was noted to generate an electric charge. Application of an oscillating current across the crystal resulted in contraction and expansion of the crystal and the generation of sound waves that could be recorded. Their fundamental observations led to the principle of ultrasonic transducers and detectors.

The sinking of the Titanic led to an interest in the development of devices to detect underwater objects by Paul Langevin of France and the ultimate development of sonar. The observation that sonar waves killed fish provided the initial application of this technology to medicine as a therapeutic modality for tumor destruction or to heal damaged tissue. Although Karl and Friederich Dussik of Austria introduced hyperphonography in 1947 the results were dubious and George Ludwig of the USA in 1949 was the first to convincingly use the technique in diagnosis. His experimental demonstration of gallstones and foreign bodies was followed by the work of John J. Wild, who successfully distinghuished the layers of the bowel wall and differentiated malignant from benign tissue in both bowel and breast. Advances in technology allowed the development of real time scanning as well as the development of Doppler ultrasound, whereby flow could be quantified as well as tissue characterized. R. Uchida and Hiroki Watanabe introduced the "ultrasonic chair" and developed the initial internal probes that have subsequently become the basis of endoscopic ultrasonography.

The first prototype of the mechanical sector scanning instruments for endoscopic ultrasound introduced in the early 1980s displayed only 180° images. The subsequent introduction of a full 360° image endoscope, the Olympus GF-UM3, provided the first commercially available echo endoscope, although there were few with adequate expertise to utilize it. Initially designed to facilitate ultrasound imaging of the pancreas, EUS has become extremely useful in the staging of gastrointestinal cancers, the identification of intramural lesions and the determination of the nature of intramural masses. In addition the development of EUS directed fine needle aspiration (FNA) cytology has enabled this technique to become an important tool in the staging of gastrointestinal cancer.

The current types of EUS equipment include 1) radial scanning; 2) curved linear array (CLA) echo endoscopes; 3) catheter based ultrasound probes. The curved linear array echo endoscope possesses an ultrasound transducer fundamentally different from that of the mechanical sector scanning endoscope in that it consists of multiple small piezo-ceramic elements mounted in a rectangular configuration on a curved surface. Electronic activation of these elements provides a pie shaped image, which radiates out perpendicularly from the transducer. Advantages of such instruments are that they can support pulse and color Doppler functions as well as FNA. Since the needle is maintained in the plane of the ultrasound image real time imaging of the tip enables a CLA endoscope to be utilized for diagnostic or therapeutic management of extramural structures. The application of EUS for both FNA as well as efficient imaging requires the development of a hybrid instrument with both radial and linear orientation. This requires a phased array transducer in the configuration of a ring combined with a rectangular phased array transducer oriented in line with the biopsy channel of the echo endoscope

The most widely used instrument is the mechanical sector scanning endoscope (Olympus Optical, Tokyo, Japan) which possesses dual frequency capability and consists of latex balloon surrounding the transducer, which can be filled with water by depressing an air water button. Since it possesses four-direction tip control it can be used for imaging within the esophagus, stomach, duodenum (pancreas and biliary tree) and the rectum. The nature of the transducer, however, prohibits the use of pulse or color Doppler functions and EUS directed FNA is difficult with this model.

The availability of catheter based ultrasound probes has amplified the utility of EUS and the use of "over the wire" versions facilitated usage in the pancreatico-biliary tree. Catheter probes provide excellent images of the GI tract wall and can identify lesions of 1-2mm in diameter. The down side of the technology is the need to connect the catheters to a motor drive as well as to a standard ultrasound processor.

Acquisition of EUS imagery has greatly advanced the staging of gastrointestinal cancer since it is in most circumstances more effective than CT scanning, although enhanced modalities (helical CT and MRI) may provide more information and are less invasive. It is possible that endoluminal magnetic resonance imaging might be useful, but this technology has yet to be applied to endoscopy.

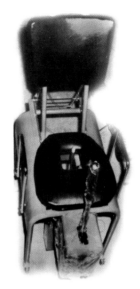

Although the first rectal transducer probes had been designed by J. Wild in the early 1950's, H. Watanabe of Japan in 1974 devised the "ultrasonic chair", in which transrectal ultrasonography could be undertaken by inserting a scanner through a hole in the seat.

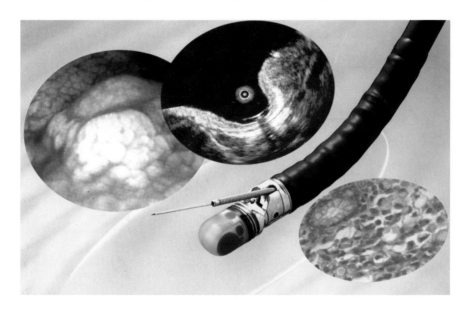

A state of the art (c. 2000) endoscopic ultrasound device with fine needle aspirator. The visual image of the lesion is at left and the ultrasonographic image is center. The fine needle aspirate is shown bottom right.

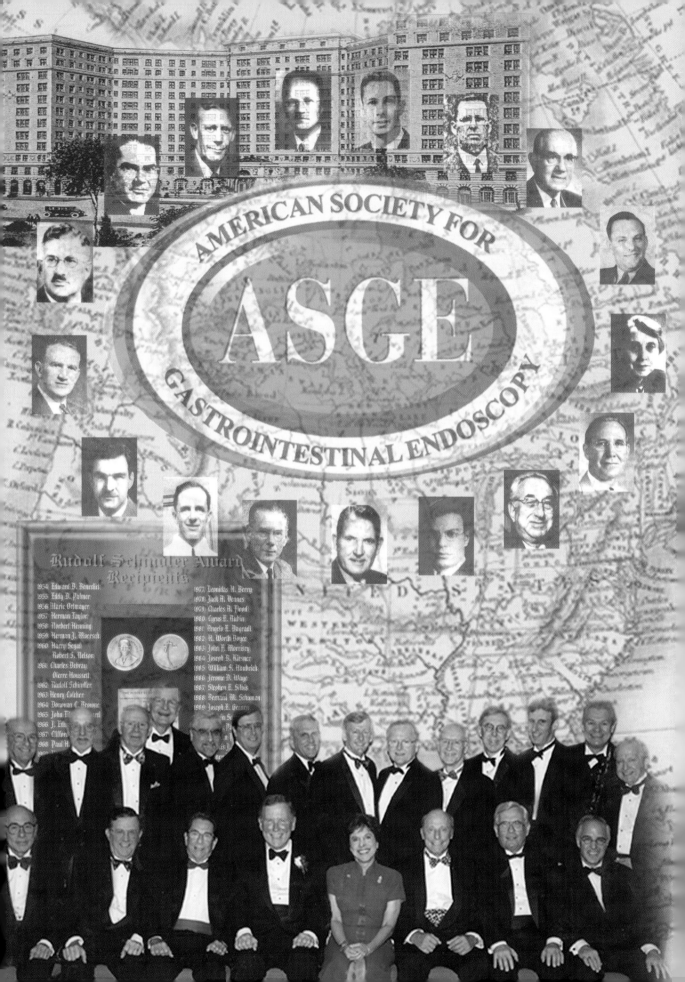

AMERICAN SOCIETY FOR

ASGE

GASTROINTESTINAL ENDOSCOPY

Rudolf Schindler Award
Recipients

1954 Edward B. Benedict
1955 Eddy D. Palmer
1956 Marie Ortmayer
1957 Herman Taylor
1958 Norbert Henning
1959 Herman J. Moersch
1960 Harry Segal
        Robert S. Nelson
1961 Charles Debray
        Pierre Houssett
1962 Rudolf Schindler
1963 Henry Colcher
1964 Donovan C. Browne
1965 John T. Howard
1966 J. Edward
1967 Clifford
1968 Paul H.

1977 Leonidas H. Berry
1978 Jack A. Vennes
1979 Charles R. Flood
1980 Cyrus E. Rubin
1981 Angelo E. Dagradi
1982 H. Worth Boyce
1983 John F. Morrissey
1984 Joseph B. Kirsner
1985 William S. Haubrich
1986 Jerome D. Waye
1987 Stephen E. Silvis
1988 Bernard M. Schuman
1989 Joseph E. Geenen

ENDOSCOPIC
SOCIETIES

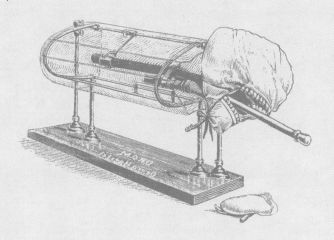

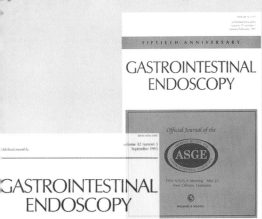

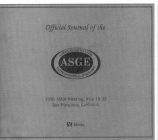

THE SCHINDLER - SCHIFF INITIATIVE

Although there had been an ongoing interest in gastroscopy in the United States since the beginning of the century, Schindler's arrival in Chicago in 1934 provided the critical momentum in its development. In this respect his meeting in 1924 with Marie Ortmayer and Grant Laing of the University of Chicago in Munich proved most propitious in that their mutual interest in endoscopy facilitated the development of a both a personal and professional friendship. Thus when Schindler was incarcerated in Dachau, Ortmayer in particular was most helpful in facilitating his immigration to the United States and arranging a medical staff position at the University of Chicago under the Chairmanship of Walter Palmer.

Although Schindler's impact on endoscopy in the United States has been previously discussed in detail, it is necessary to briefly reiterate some of the details within the perspective of the development of the American Society for Gastro Intestinal Endoscopy. During the first five years in America it became apparent to Schindler as well as a number of his colleagues interested in gastroenterology that gastroscopy had not been accepted as an important part of gastroenterology. Indeed the meetings of the American Gastroenterology Association (AGA) had failed to provide the needed forum for the subject and in addition the American Medical Association (AMA) was not particularly supportive.

Leon Schiff of the University of Cincinnati (*top*) and John Renshaw of the Cleveland Clinic (*bottom*) proposed late in 1940 that a meeting should be held in June of 1941 at the Cleveland Clinic to establish a Gastroscopic Society. Although Schindler initially supported this idea, he subsequently withdrew declaring that such a group should not convene before appropriate diplomatic groundwork had been laid with the diverse array of relevant medical organizations. The first meeting was therefore postponed until November of 1941 and held in Chicago at Schindler's residence.

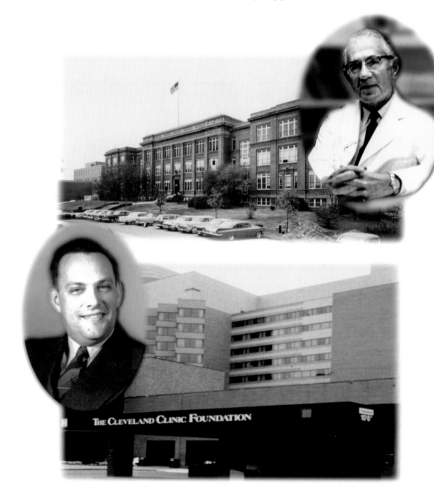

Late in 1940 and during the early part of 1941, Leon Schiff of the University of Cincinnati had suggested to several individuals in the United States interested in gastroscopy that a gastroscopic society be formed. It was proposed that a meeting under the sponsorship of John Renshaw be undertaken in June of 1941 at the Cleveland Clinic to consolidate this proposal. Although Schindler was initially a proponent of this idea, he subsequently withdrew his support since he was concerned that such a society might be viewed as establishing gastroscopy as a separate specialty and thus limit its use rather than expand its availability.

The Foundation of the Club

In mid-February of 1941 Schindler therefore formally communicated to his colleagues that he was against the proposed Cleveland meeting and suggested that it be canceled until appropriate groundwork with the different societies had been undertaken. It was therefore agreed upon that the meeting be postponed until Schindler had contacted the various relevant organizations. He formally communicated with the American College of Surgeons, the American College of Physicians, the American Board of Internal Medicine, the American Board of Surgery, the AGA, and the Sections of Internal Medicine, Surgery, and Gastroenterology and Proctology of the American Medical Association to assure them that the meeting was not an attempt to establish gastroscopy as a distinct and separate specialty. As a result of having successfully undertaken the necessary groundwork over the next 3 months, it was agreed by all that the initial exploratory meeting should be scheduled to take place in Chicago in November 1941. On September the 11th, 1941, Schindler distributed a carefully drafted letter to a number of individuals who he perceived would be interested in forming a gastroscopic society.

Since funding was an issue, Schindler proposed that the meeting be held in his apartment and that if it was concluded that no organization was necessary, the group should adjourn to the nearby Windermere Hotel three blocks from his apartment where a good dinner could be had for $1-$1.50. Alternatively, if the participants decided that an organization might be of merit, the dinner could be dispensed with in favor of drafting a constitution, developing bylaws, electing a governing board, and

A meeting to decide whether a gastroscopic society should be established took place on November 9, 1941 at Schindler's home in Chicago. At the end of an afternoon of heated discussion, all participants agreed that they perceived merit in the idea and repaired to the adjacent Windermere Hotel (*top*) for a celebratory dinner. The salubrious dining room of the hotel (*center*) offered a gourmet repast (*bottom right*, *1941 menu*) for a modest $1-1.50 and the 17 founding members were no doubt well satisfied at the accomplishments of the day. Although no details of the exact wine list can be traced, rumor holds that the cheese (*bottom left*) was taken with a Chateau Maligny, L'Homme Mort 1934 to dispel the premonitions of E.F. Sauerbruch.

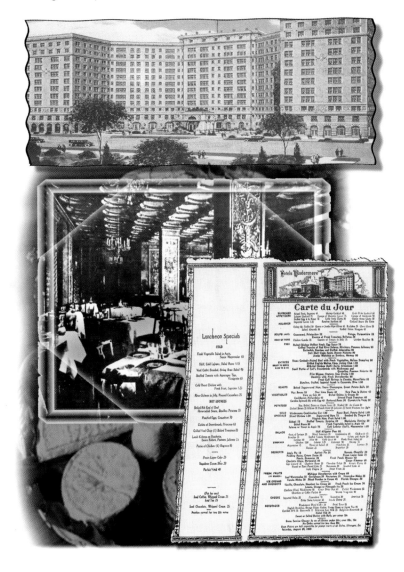

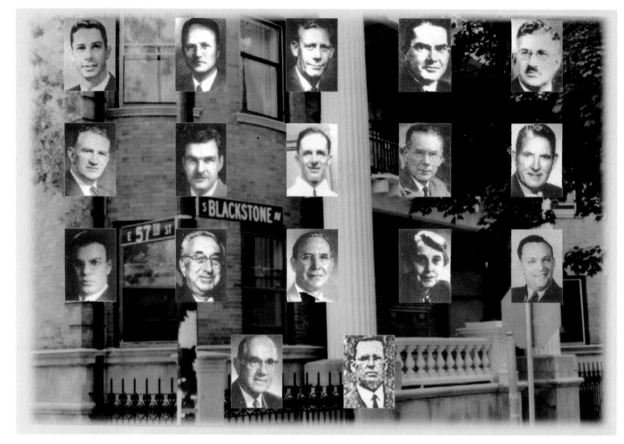

The birth of the American Gastroscopic Club (AGC) took place at R. Schindler's Chicago home, 5608 Blackstone Av. (*background*) Nov. 9th, 1941 at 2.30 p.m. Those present included *from left to right, top row*: C.F. Barnett, E.B. Benedict, J. Borland Sr., J.B. Carey, A.L. Cohn; *2nd row*: J.H. Fitzgibbon, C.A. Flood, R. Schindler, J.T. Howard, R.H. Keane; *3rd row*: B. Kenamore, J.B. Kirsner, H.J. Moersch, M Ortmayer, J F. Renshaw; *4th row*: Leon Schiff and Ray Sexton. In an attempt to safeguard the external concept that gastroscopy might be regarded as a specialty in the making, it was agreed by all present that consideration should be given to dissolving the society as soon as its goals were achieved!

other appropriate administrative issues. On October 14 a second letter containing the agenda for the meeting was sent to potential participants. Edward Benedict of Boston, who was widely regarded as a major protagonist of gastroscopy, was asked by Schindler to speak against the concept of advancing the gastroscopic method and thereby provide the basis for an open debate. Other members were asked to address issues such as the teaching of gastroscopy, the construction and design of gastroscopes and the relationship of the subject to gastroenterology in general.

The First Meeting

On November 9, 1941 at 2:30 p.m. the first meeting of the fledgling endoscopy group (17 individuals) took place at Schindler's home in 5608 Blackstone Avenue near the University of Chicago.

Those present included R. Schindler, Crawford F. Barnett (Atlanta), Edward B. Benedict (Boston), James Borland (Jacksonville, Florida), James B. Carey (Minneapolis), Allan L. Cohn (San Francisco), John H. Fitzgibbon (Portland, Oregon), Charles A. Flood (New York City), John T. Howard (Baltimore), Roger Keane (Portland, Oregon), Bruce Kenamore (St. Louis), Joseph B. Kirsner (Chicago), Herman J. Moersch (Rochester, Minnesota), Marie Ortmayer (Chicago), John F. Renshaw (Cleveland), Leon Schiff (Cincinnati) and Roy Sexton (Washington, D.C.). The opening discussion of the meeting featured a "debate" between Schindler and Benedict as to whether there was any need for such a society.

Benedict proposed that the existence of a society would lead to over specialization and isolation, but Schindler argued that the state of gastroscopy in the United States was deteriorating since the technique and its utility were not only misunderstood, but for the most part undertaken by individuals without appropriate training. He was particularly concerned that it was becoming regarded as a mere technical procedure and that there was little recognition of the fact that sophisticated interpretation requiring both specialized technical and diagnostic skills was required.

Apart from his focus on the role that the society might play in the broader context of American medicine, Schindler was particularly interested in the use of gastroscopy to identify the source of gastric complaints for which no overt organic pathology could be demonstrated. It was his belief that dyspeptic disease in the army and navy was a major health consideration and its appropriate diagnosis and treatment critical to the maintenance of the morale of the fighting forces. Over the course of many subsequent years Schindler persevered with the health of the armed forces, and sought diligently to both identify the precise nature of gastritis and develop an appropriate therapeutic strategy for its treatment. Much of his subsequent writing would focus on the issue of gastritis and indeed his obsession with the subject would lead to a serious clash with Walter Palmer, his chairman, who perceived little merit in Schindler's observations.

After some hours of discussion it became apparent to the participants that a general consensus existed in support of the formation of an organization. At this stage debate rose at to what it should be named. Among the suggestions entertained were "The Association of Gastroscopy", "Association for the Advancement of Gastroscopy", "American Gastroscopic Research Organization" and "American Gastroscopic Society". Although Schindler favored the latter, the majority of his colleagues believed that the word "club" should be used since it was less pretentious. Sensitive to the associations of the word ""club" in his native Germany, Schindler believed that this title lacked dignity. Nevertheless, the proposal by James Brolin that the organization adopt the title of "The American Gastroscopic Club" was seconded by Ortmayer and thereupon accepted by the group. Schiff cast no votes since he favored an informal discussion group and Renshaw abstained with the result that the motion carried by six votes. In the aftermath of the vote Schindler was elected President, Benedict vice president, and Joseph Kirsner the Secretary Treasurer.

The meeting thereupon adjourned for dinner at the Windmere Hotel and in the early evening the group returned to the apartment where Schindler entertained them with his piano playing skills and others sang selections from Gilbert and Sullivan operettas.

Dr. Joseph B. Kirsner, (*center*) a founding member of American Gastroscopic Club (AGC) exemplifies the caliber of the individuals who participated in its establishment. Elected secretary treasurer at its first meeting in 1941, he had by the turn of the century not only participated in the founding of almost all the major American societies devoted to digestive disease, but been President of both the AGA and the AGC. As a recipient of the Rudolf Schindler Award (ASGE), Friedenwald Medal (AGA), John Phillips Memorial Award (ACP), George Howell Coleman Medal (Institute of Medicine of Chicago), the Gold key Award and the Alumni Medal of the University of Chicago (*background*), he became a gastroenterologic legend in his own lifetime.

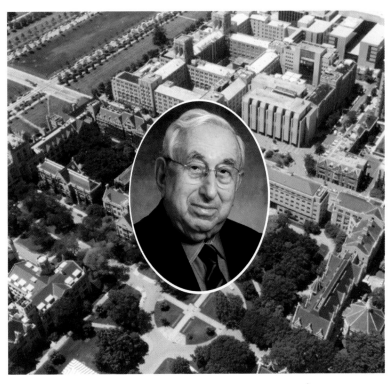

THE EARLY DAYS

On June 7, 1942, when the first meeting of the fledgling American Gastroscopic Club was held at the Hotel Claridge in Atlantic City, its membership had grown to 109. The rationale for the timing reflected the fact that most members were gastroenterologists and to facilitate travel the club therefore convened a day after the AGA meeting. As the first president of the club it was Schindler's prerogative to choose the topic and as might have been predicted he proposed that gastritis be the order of the day. Thus the first scientific session consisting of seven papers on gastritis was entitled *"Symposium on Symptomatology of Chronic Gastritis with Special Reference to the Conditions in the Army and the Navy"*. Although Walter Alvarez, the editor of the *American Journal of Digestive Diseases*, had been approached by Schindler to publish the symposium, this arrangement failed to materialize and the transactions of the first meeting were subsequently published in *Gastroenterology*, the newly established journal of the American Gastroenterology Association.

A week after the first meeting of the club a second informal meeting to discuss membership requirements was held in Chicago immediately after the American Medical Association meeting. Despite the absence of Schindler and thus without a president, a number of important areas were developed by those present. The first dealt with the question of membership requirements. Thus the Articles of Association stated that every member should be a physician, have adequate training in gastroscopy, be a member of a scientific organizations of recognized standards, or be approved as a specialist in gastroenterology, internal medicine, or surgery and file an application with the society accompanied by recommendations from two members. The second issue discussed was that of standards of training and those present agreed that a committee (M. Ortmayer, H.M. Pollard from Ann Arbor and Leo L. Hardt from Chicago) be established to determine appropriate standards.

In order to facilitate interaction with the general membership, a newsletter entitled *Bulletin of the American Gastroscopic Club* was first published in September, 1942. Despite its modest size (4 pages) and its somewhat amateur nature, it proved

The first scientific meeting of the American Gastroscopic Club (109 members) was held on June 7, 1942 at the Hotel Claridge (*far right*) adjacent to the balmy boardwalk of Atlantic City, New Jersey, a day after the AGA meeting. R. Schindler, the first President, organized a scientific program (*left*) that consisted of seven papers dealing with his special area of interest, namely the relevance of chronic gastritis in members of the military services.

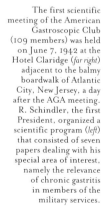

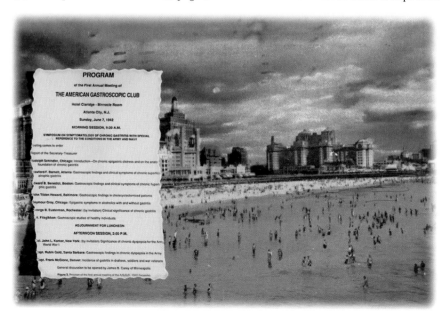

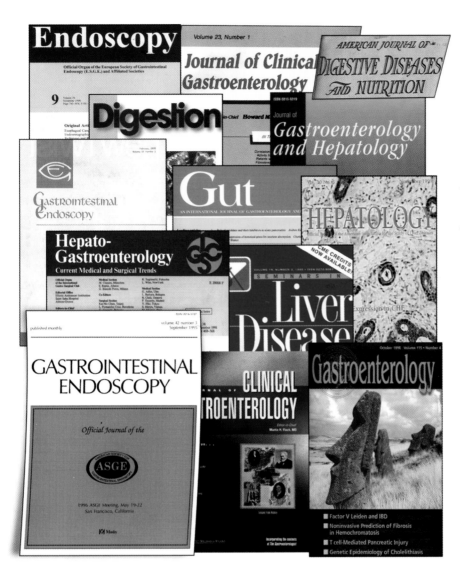

The first journal devoted entirely to the subject of gastroenterology, *Die Archiv der Verdauungskrankenheiten*, was founded and edited by I. Boas in Berlin in 1896. Although at the turn of the 19th century only one journal was available, over the next two decades this would increase to four or five and by the end of the 20th century a diverse array of gastrointestinal journals were available. Since the fledgling American Gastroscopic Club possessed no formal journal, it published the proceedings of its first scientific meeting in a newly established journal, *Gastroenterology*, which was the official organ of the AGA. In order to expand its visibility and further interact with its members it thereafter in September of 1942 began publishing, albeit intermittently, a four-page newsletter entitled *Bulletin of the American Gastroscopic Club*. Over the next 50 years this modest periodical would metamorphasize into an internationally recognized journal and stern arbiter of endoscopic progress.

to be both an important tool in allowing the membership to remain in contact with each other as well as providing information regarding club news, case reports, and military concerns. As the sole editor, Schindler was responsible for its production and by dint of hard work ensured that it appeared twice a year usually in January and June. Despite having been the catalytic agent in American gastroscopy, the path taken by Schindler was not as smooth as might have been predicted or wished for and his tenure as President of the Gastroscopic Club terminated in 1943 consequent upon his abrupt departure from Chicago. Although still an active participant in the activities of the club, Schindler was succeeded by Edward Benedict as President in 1943.

By 1944 the club had convened a committee on teaching standards and more than 100 questionnaires were sent out to solicit information on current teaching practices in gastroscopy. It was concluded that proper training with the right facility should include "observations of at least 50 cases, knowledge of indications and contraindications, practical technique and interpretation." Although informal meetings of the officers or the governing board continued on an *ad hoc* basis, the Second World War obviated further meetings of the club until June of 1945, when the second annual meeting of the club was once again held in Atlantic City immediately after the AGA meeting. Given the interest of the President (Benedict) in surgical gastroscopy and biopsy, the program was entitled "*The Differential Diagnosis of Benign and Malignant Lesions of the Stomach*" and was discussed from the perspective of pathologists, gastroscopists, clinicians and radiologists. Although no formal arrangements had been undertaken to publish the presentations of 1945, it was agreed that papers read at the next annual meeting should all be submitted to *Gastroenterology*, and as a result three articles were published in 1946.

In the same year the membership of the club also decided that the *Bulletin* should be upgraded and the first editor, H. Marvin Pollard and an associate editor Roy Sexton were elected. Within two years it was proposed that the *Bulletin* be amplified and a debate ensued as to whether this required either more issues or that each issue be larger. Consequently the *Bulletin* continued biannually but expanded in size with increased numbers of scientific articles to become six to eight pages per

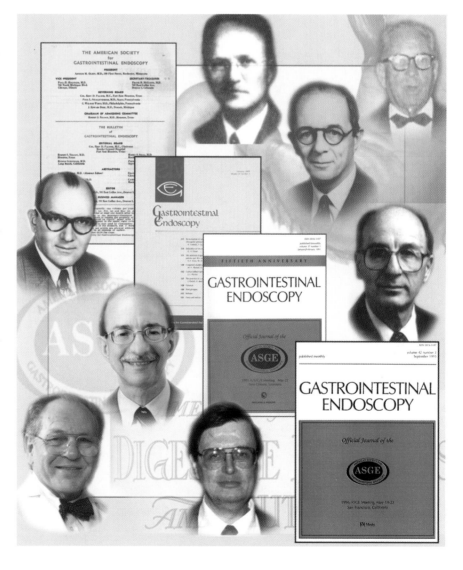

The *Bulletin* evolved from a modest, intermittently published newsletter edited initially by R. Schindler (*center right oblique*) and thereafter by E. Benedict (*top right oblique*) to a formal scientific journal, *Gastrointestinal Endoscopy*. The first editor was H. Marvin Pollard (*extreme left center*), who was succeeded by Roy Sexton in 1957. Thereafter Col. Horace Marvin and Walter Palmer (1961) played a major role in amplifying the journal size and publication numbers. The appointment of William Haubrich (1971) (*bottom left*) presaged an era of unprecedented growth and popularity of the journal. Thereafter Bernard Schuman (1981) (*extreme right center*), Charles J.Lightdale (1989) (*center of the left oblique*) and M. Sivak (1997) (*center bottom*) each played a substantial role in establishing the journal at the forefront of the field of endoscopy. A former President of the society, John Tilden Howard (*top right*), in 1970 assumed a somewhat more lighthearted editorial role by publishing an article entitled the "*Gospel of Gastroscopy in the United States*".

issue. Over a period of eight years the *Bulletin* evolved from a newsletter type publication to a more formal clinical and scientific journal. After five years of productive management, Pollard relinquished his editorial responsibilities in 1951 and Roy Sexton assumed this role for the following decade.

FROM CLUB TO SOCIETY

In 1947 the club voted to change its name to "American Gastroscopic Society" in deference to the original wishes of Schindler. In addition they successfully petitioned the AGA to permit four or five papers to be presented at the AGA meeting itself. This proposal was accepted by the membership of the Gastroscopic Society on condition that the papers be identified as having been sponsored by the American Gastroscopic Society itself. In order to facilitate the adoption of this arrangement for the 1948 meeting in Atlantic City, a statement was prepared and sent to the AGA: "The American Gastroscopic Society accepts your suggestion that papers sponsored by the program committee of the American Gastroscopic Society be submitted to American Gastroenterological Association for con-

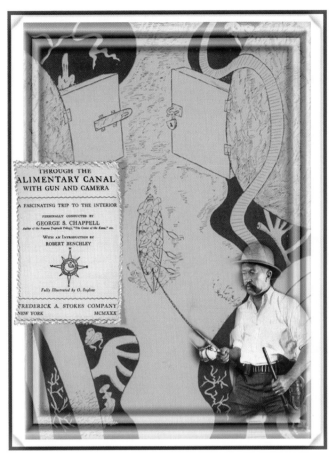

sideration for your 1949 program. It is the desire of the society that these papers be presented as a unified program." Despite the opinion of James Brolin, the President of the AGS, that a unified program at the AGA was impossible, both societies were committed to combining their meetings and despite objections, the 1949 scientific session of the AGS was incorporated into the AGA meeting and five papers presented.

As a result of this success discussions were entertained as to whether the two societies should merge and whether the *Bulletin* should be replaced by a section of gastroscopy in *Gastroenterology*. Although the latter proposal met with some support given the difficulty in obtaining appropriate publishable gastroscopic material for the *Bulletin*, the issue of a societal merger was more vexatious. Indeed so strong were the feelings supporting amalgamation of the two societies that in 1950 a committee representing both organizations was convened to formally discuss this issue. Consequent upon these deliberations it was proposed that the societies merge. The recommendations included in the merger suggested the establishment of a committee on endoscopy within the AGA as well as the issuance of an invitation to gastroscopic society members to participate fully in the AGA. While these suggestions were well accepted, the additional proposal that the funds of the Gastroscopic Society be turned over to the AGA and utilized for furthering the purposes of endoscopy, education and research in gastroenterology, failed to excite acclamation or engender enthusiasm. Indeed the latter issue proved to be the "deal breaker" and after vigorous discussion, it was decided by the membership of the Society that they should pursue their own aspirations.

G. Chappell published a book, *"Through the Alimentary Canal with Gun and Camera"*, that entertained a less serious viewpoint of gastrointestinal endoscopy.

In 1950, Julian Buser, under the guidance of Joseph Kirsner, produced a noteworthy issue that contained a comprehensive list of 501 articles and books on gastroscopy published between 1934 and 1949. A thousand copies were published and mailed to every hospital and medical library in the country.

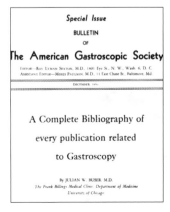

THE ISSUE OF TRAINING REQUIREMENTS

By the end of the first decade of its existence a number of issues faced the society. These included: 1) the relationship with the AGA; 2) the establishment of standards of training; 3) the need to ensure adequate quality of instrumentation; and 4) the question of the development of standards and guidelines by which practitioners could be judged competent to undertake endoscopy. This latter area was particularly vexatious and had also been addressed by the American College of Surgeons, the American Hospital Association, and the American Medical Association. The concept of control of standards of practice was complex and sensitive. Since it raised matters that were related to competence and patient care it also provoked debate as to the legality of privileging and the question of whether this might be interpreted or construed as restraint of trade. Lastly, the establishment of such parameters brought into debate the long revered American creed of autonomy and the sensitivities pertaining to external regulation.

As with all novel techniques, the issues related to training and ensuring competence became a vexatious issue. One of the original goals propounded by Schindler and the founders of the AGC in 1941 was the need to ensure that physicians were adequately trained in the indications for gastroscopy as well as the use of the instruments. It was soon apparent that lectures (*bottom*: 1950's meeting of the AGC) and diagrams were not adequate and that tuition in "hands on skills" were required. Utilizing techniques first employed in the early 1920's by the urologists to teach cystoscopy (bladder phantom, *right*) the pioneers of gastroscopy developed similar phantoms for the upper gastrointestinal tract (*top left*). Such teaching tools and techniques have since evolved enormously and virtual reality simulators have now supplanted the latex models of the 80's.

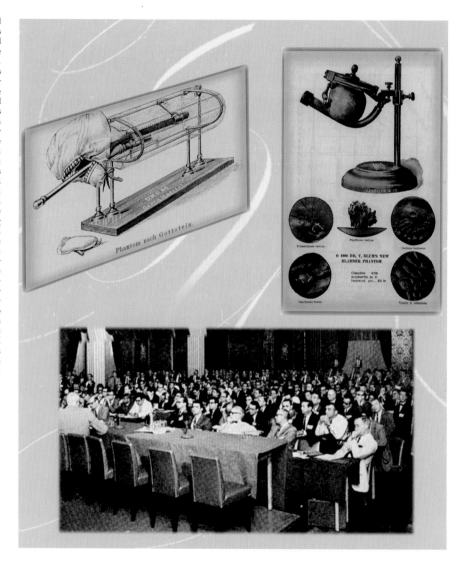

The Second and Third Decades (1951-1971)

One of the early issues of the second decade of the existence of the society was its recognition that esophagoscopy might be considered to fall within their domain of interest. In the earlier part of the century otolaryngologists had focused on the esophagus, but as gastroscopy became more prevalent among gastroenterologists, the consideration that the esophagus might fall within their sphere of expertise was raised. Indeed as early as 1946, John Tilden Howard, the secretary of the society, had been vocal in pointing out to gastroenterologists the need to examine the esophagus.

The society and its membership were of the firm opinion that none was more competent than the gastroenterologist in this area. Based upon the evolution of such sentiment and the advent of safer esophagoscopes and the increasing general access to the esophagus, the society deemed it worthy it of consideration that esophagoscopy be included as part of its mandate. The drive towards the inclusion of the esophagus in the ambit of the Society culminated in 1959 with the membership requirements being formally revised to reflect the necessity of the possession of esophagoscopic skills and in addition the amplification of the *Bulletin* title to *The Bulletin of Gastroscopy and Esophagoscopy*.

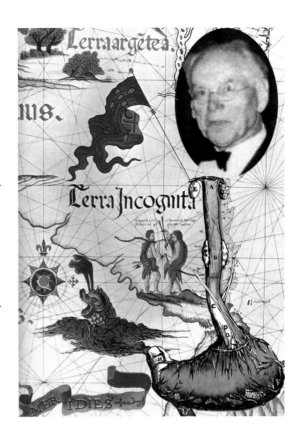

John Tilden Howard (*top right*) noted that with the advent of novel therapeutic strategies for esophageal disease it had become apparent that the esophagus could no longer be regarded as *terra incognita* or "no man's land". Although all acknowledged that the discipline of otolaryngology had pioneered esophageal endoscopy and that radiology had amplified the understanding of both its physiology and diagnosis, the question of treatment of esophageal diseases had now became pertinent. With perspicuity Tilden raised the complex issue of "domain of expertise" and urged the membership of the Society to direct its attention to the esophagus.

The decade of the 50s had not been easy times for the *Bulletin* and the new editor, Roy Sexton, had struggled to maintain both quality and quantity of content while combating fiduciary difficulties. Indeed so dire had the situation become, that in 1956 only one issue of the *Bulletin* was published and discussions were initiated with the *American Journal of Digestive Diseases* in consideration of adopting this organ as an optional publication vehicle. Although this relationship failed to materialize the scientific proceedings of the annual meeting of 1957 were published in *Gastroenterology*. Unfortunately this solution too would prove flawed since within the next year it became apparent that *Gastroenterology* could not cope with the volume of material provided by the society. The inordinate delays in publication lead to a redirection of attention to the matter of resuscitation of the *Bulletin*. In 1958 the governing board decided to amplify the support of the *Bulletin* by instituting two measures. Firstly it was decided to increase the annual number of issues to four, and secondly, to require papers presented at the annual meeting be submitted to the *Bulletin* for first consideration. By 1959 it appeared that with the added support from the society and the acquisition of some advertising revenues, the situation had been stabilized. Unfortunately the promised four issues per year could not be delivered and since the *Bulletin* had changed its name in 1959 to the *Bulletin of Gastroscopy and Esophagoscopy*, advertisers deemed that their contract was nullified. As a result of this series of setbacks, the fiscal problems of the *Bulletin* were so serious by 1960 that publication was suspended and R. Sexton resigned. Undaunted by this adversity the Society revamped the administration of the *Bulletin*, appointed a new editor, Colonel Horace Marvin, and by the end of 1961 was once again back in publication.

At the annual meeting of the society on May 16, 1957 at the Broadmoor Hotel in Colorado, Basil Hirschowitz (*center*) at the invitation of the President of the American Society for Gastroscopy, John Tilden Howard, demonstrated the utility of the fiber optic endoscope. Larry Curtiss (*top*) of Ann Arbor had collaborated with Hirschowitz in producing glass fibers for the gastroscope and wound the original sets on a "Mother Oats" cardboard box (*left*). H. Hopkins of England (*bottom*) had been responsible for the introduction of the modern concept of the use of glass fibers for light transmission. This early flexible gastroscope (*center*) was able to convey an image (*bottom*, original Lincoln stamp image, 1957) and in so doing ushered in a new era of internal vision as the semi-flexible gastroscope (*right*) was supplanted. Hirschowitz's presentation was received with modest enthusiasm little different to the relatively cool reception accorded to Antonin J. Desormeaux by the Parisian *Academie des Sciences* on November 29, 1855 after his demonstration of the first truly functional endoscope. Although much had changed in the ensuing century, men had obviously changed little!

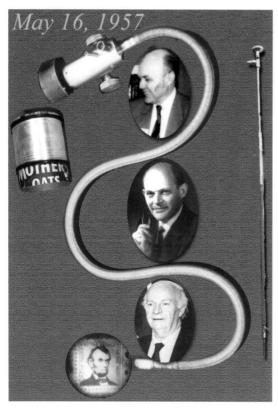

May 16, 1957

The Fiber and the Future

At the annual meeting of the society at the Broadmoor Hotel in Colorado Springs in 1957 the entire world of endoscopy would be changed. The President, John Tilden Howard, announced "at half past eight o'clock Dr. Hirschowitz will tell you about what I understand to be a new principle of gastroscopy. I hear that fiberglass conducts light around corners and that Dr. H. has used this material in a new type of gastroscope…". A diminutive audience of approximately 40 persons witnessed the demonstration and presentation at 8:30 a.m. of Hirschowitz's prototype instrument.

Despite the fact that they had witnessed the dawn of a new era, the response was muted and even as late as 1961 the minutes of the society's governing board meeting would cautiously note that "…although the board recognized the importance of this new development in the field of endoscopy, it was recommended that the board encourage its members to continue gastroscopy with standard instruments and await further developments…". This conservatism was supported by the rationale that it was the skill of the gastroscopists themselves and not the technology of the instrumentation which would determine the success and effectiveness of the technique. Nevertheless, the advancing role of technology coupled with the intrinsic creativity of various members of the society led to the advent of the gastric camera and the gastro-camera fiberoscope within a relatively short period of time. In 1961 Eddy Palmer, the president of the society, could state with some degree of pride that what had formerly been a Gastroscopy Society had evolved not only into an Esophagogastroscopic Society, but had now transmogrified itself into a Panendoscopy Society. As a consequence of such exhortations, the membership elected to once again alter the name of the society to the "American Society for Gastrointestinal Endoscopy" and with this emmendation to in addition revise the *Bulletin* title to the *Bulletin of Gastrointestinal Endoscopy*.

The Expansion of Horizons

Having begun as a modest group of seventeen indivduals in a small downtown apartment in Chicago, the society had over 20 years achieved a position of considerable influence and responsibility. Not only was its national status widely recognized, but in 1958 its active participation in the World Congress of Gastroenterology in Washington D.C confirmed its attainment of international visibility. As a result of the establishment of an informal relationship with the European Endoscopic Club (EEC) in 1960, a joint meeting was undertaken at the following World Congress of Gastroenterology held in Munich in 1962. Similarly the society played an active role in planning the first International Meeting of Gastrointestinal Endoscopy held in Tokyo in 1966 and appointed J. Edward Burke as its representative to coordinate the selection of papers to be presented from North and South America.

In addition to amplifying its international presence at national level meetings, educational issues were deemed to be of paramount importance, and in 1962 a symposium entitled

"Teaching Methods in Gastrointestinal Endoscopy" was held in New York City. Indeed this topic was considered to be so fundamental to the function of the society, that in 1964 the president, Paul H. Holinger (an otolarygologist), established a committee to establish the minimum requirements for training endoscopists. It concluded that three issues were necessary: 1) a full training in medicine or surgery that covered all fundamental areas pertaining to disorders of the gastrointestinal tract; 2) additional and special training in all aspects of gastrointestinal endoscopy under the supervision of an acceptable instructor; 3) observation and performance of an adequate number of gastrointestinal endoscopic procedures. It is worthy of note that the committee also went on record as stating that such training should be regarded as an integral part of all training programs in gastroenterology. To further these aims, the society thereafter established its own training program and in May 1966, offered the first post graduate training course at the Cook County Hospital in Chicago. This initial venture proved to be most successful and by 1969 had been established as a integral annual component of the activity of the society.

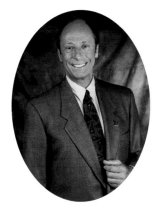

Melvin Schapiro, President of the ASGE (1984–5), facilitated the educational and scientific activities of the society at both a national and international level.

World Organization for Digestive Endoscopy (OMED)

Given the mounting international interest in the subject a number of endoscopic societies were founded. Based upon mutual agreement it was agreed that such groups should be established based upon their geographic location and three global zones were therefore created. The Asian-Pacific Society was established in 1966, the European in 1968 and the Inter American in 1973. Their success led to the consideration of initiating a central coordinating group charged with the responsibility of providing international oversight and coordination of endoscopy on a worldwide basis.

Thus at the 2nd World Congress of Gastroenterology held in Munich in 1962, Drs. Tasaka, Hayashida, Yamagata, Masuda, Sakita and others, proposed the creation of an International Society of Endoscopy (ISE). It was further agreed that the members of the Japanese Committee, under the guidance of Dr. Masuda would accept the responsibility of drafting a constitution for this group. Two years later at the European Congress of Gastroenterology in Brussels the draft was approved and the ISE inaugurated.

At this early stage, since the ISE had no financial support it was necessary to hold its first meetings in conjunction with the World Congress of Gastroenterology. In 1966 over 700 participants attended the 1st World Congress of Digestive Endoscopy in Tokyo under the presidency of Dr. Tasaka.

In 1973 at the Pan American Congress of Gastroenterology held in Buenos Aires a final decision was made to organize a World Society that would include the three zones of the Asian-Pacific, the Inter-American and the European. The International Society of Digestive Endoscopy was thus established in Mexico City in October, 1974 and in 1975 at the meeting of the Vice-Presidents held in Caracas, Venezuela, it altered its name to World Organization for Digestive Endoscopy (O.M.E.D.). Although in its early years OMED was a "token" representative at the planning committee of the World Congresses of São Paulo (1986) and Sydney

In 1998 at the World Congress of Gastroenterology and Digestive Endoscopy held in Vienna a new governing board was empowered for a 4 years term (1998-2002): Glaciomar Machado, Brazil (President) (*center*), Alexandre Abrao-Neto, Brazil (Secretary-General) (*absent*), Jerome D. Waye, USA (Treasurer) (*right*) and Hirohumi Niwa, Japan (President-elect) (*left*).

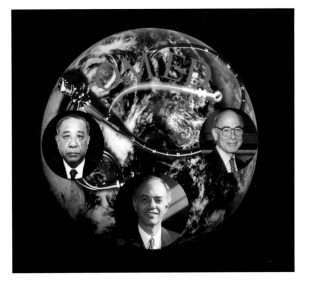

(1990), by 1994 at Los Angeles, OMED had begun to exert an international influence in the organization of the meeting.

Individuals who each have made great contributions to the development of endoscopy have ably served the society. Its presidents have included Sadataka Tasaka (Japan), Henry Colcher (USA), Wilfrid Sircus (UK), Horacio Rubio (Argentina), Klaus Heinkel (FRG); Masasuke Masuda (Japan), Takao, Sakita (Japan), Rodolfo Cheli (Italy) and Massimo Crespi (Italy). At this time, OMED is fully recognized as an independent society, representing endoscopy at a worldwide level by encouraging and stimulating close cooperation and interchange between the Organization and the 3 international zones. Its main activities include the Education Committee (dissemination of the OMED endoscopy training program), the Research Committee (promotion of International Cooperative studies), Terminology Committee (establishment of a worldwide iminimal standard terminology) for data processing in digestive endoscopy.

SCHINDLER AND THE SOCIETY

Despite the fact that Schindler was the founding father of the society, the relationship between he and the society had fluctuated in the early years after his departure from the University of Chicago. A number of overtures and attempts to re-establish a mutually productive relationship had not met with success and an uncomfortable situation remained. Despite this state of affairs, the society sought to honor Schindler and in October 1953 the Schindler Award was established at the suggestion of Joseph Kirsner, who had proposed that an award to recognize outstanding achievement in gastroscopy be considered.

In 1954 Marie Ortmayer, an old and dear friend of Schindler, was elected President of the society, but even her presence failed to completely mollify Schindler and although he continued to maintain a cordial relationship with the society it was distant. Unfortunately in 1960 the fragile association once again deteriorated consequent upon a dispute relating to a manuscript submitted by Schindler for publication. Nevertheless, mutual generosity of spirit prevailed and in 1962 Schindler himself was honored by the society as the recipient of the Schindler Award. His demise in 1968 in Munich marked the closure of a chapter in the evolution of the society. Irrespective of the turbulent nature of

The Rudolf Schindler award was established in 1953 at the suggestion of Joseph Kirsner. The list of awardees ranging from Edward Benedict (1954) to David Fleischer (2000) represents the acknowledgement of the Society of outstanding contributions of an individual to endoscopy. The names enshrined on this plaque document the pioneers of the field over a period of half a century and memorialize in perpetuity not only their achievements but the spirit and vision of Rudolf Schindler.

Rudolf Schindler Award Recipients

1954 Edward B. Benedict	1977 Leonidas H. Berry
1955 Eddy D. Palmer	1978 Jack A. Vennes
1956 Marie Ortmayer	1979 Charles A. Flood
1957 Herman Taylor	1980 Cyrus E. Rubin
1958 Norbert Henning	1981 Angelo E. Dagradi
1959 Herman J. Moersch	1982 H. Worth Boyce
1960 Harry Segal	1983 John F. Morrisey
Robert S. Nelson	1984 Joseph B. Kirsner
1961 Charles Debray	1985 William S. Haubrich
Pierre Houssett	1986 Jerome D. Waye
1962 Rudolf Schindler	1987 Stephen E. Silvis
1963 Henry Colcher	1988 Bernard M. Schuman
1964 Donovan C. Browne	1989 Joseph E. Geenen
1965 John Tilden Howard	1990 Melvin Schapiro
1966 J. Edward Berk	1991 Joel F. Panish
1967 Clifford Barborka	1992 J. Loren Pitcher
1968 Paul H. Holinger	1993 Francis J. Tedesco
1969 Horace P. Marvin	1994 Sidney J. Winawer
1970 G. Gordon McHardy	1995 Walter J. Hogan
1971 Frank E. McGlone	1996 Glen A. Lehman
1972 Joseph P. Belber	1997 Michael V. Sivak Jr.
1973 Basil I. Hirschowitz	1998 John H. Bond
1974 Benjamin H. Sullivan	1999 Charles J. Lightdale
1975 Bergein F. Overholt	2000 David Fleischer
1976 Marvin Pollard	

THE RUDOLF SCHINDLER AWARD
THE AMERICAN SOCIETY FOR GASTROINTESTINAL ENDOSCOPY
AWARD TO
Edward B. Benedict, M.D.
ITS HIGHEST DISTINCTION
IN RECOGNITION OF OUTSTANDING CONTRIBUTIONS
TO GASTROINTESTINAL ENDOSCOPY
1954

AMERICAN SOCIETY FOR ASGE GASTROINTESTINAL ENDOSCOPY

the interaction, there can be little doubt that his contributions to both gastroscopy and the founding of the Gastroscopy Club were seminal in the evolution of the society.

The Corridors of Power: 1971–1981

This decade was characterized both by expansion and the need to establish a visible presence within the pantheon of the different digestive disease groups now vying for visibility and funding on the national scene. The Digestive Disease Week, though overcrowded, was extremely effective in allowing for the complex interface of numerous societies all focused on diseases of the gastrointestinal tract. Although the administrative arrangements for the meeting had been placed in the hands of Charles Slack and associates, there continued to be tension between the AGA and ASGE as to the governance of the meeting itself. The matter was further accentuated by the establishment of new groups including the "American Digestive Disease Society" (1972) and the "Federation of Digestive Disease Societies". Complex issues surrounding the interface of these various groups as well as their funding led to difficulties in cooperation despite an interest in the common goal of furthering the public recognition of digestive disease

In an attempt to expand its influence, the society embarked upon a reconfiguration of its internal structure to encompass and better serve the growing number of endoscopists in the country. As a result, the first regional societies were established in 1973 with southern California leading the way. Representation from such societies at a national level was effective in that it provided not only a degree of autonomy but also facilitated broad representation. This enabled the development of combined educational and research programs and the establishment of the Council of Regional Endoscopic Societies in 1974. By 1976 the initial group of seven regional societies had expanded to 25 regional groups and begun to provide widespread representation at a national level.

Seeking to ensure appropriate representation, the President of the society, Henry Colcher, in 1973 unsuccessfully requested that the ASGE be placed on the AMA Inter Specialty council. This overture reflected the complex interface between the issue of accreditation and the eligibility to receive Medicare/Medicaid payments. By establishing such representation the ASGE sought to assure the application of proper endoscopic standards to the peer review process. Unfortunately this petition was denied and the ASGE was forced to submit its guidelines directly to the AMA. Since the AGA had separately and independently submitted its own guidelines, an uncomfortable debate regarding the issue of "setting standards" arose. This culminated with the President of the AGA formerly asking Bergein F. Overholt the chairman of the ASGE Committee on Standards whether it was appropriate for any society to set such guidelines. As a result of such discussions it was proposed that a doc-

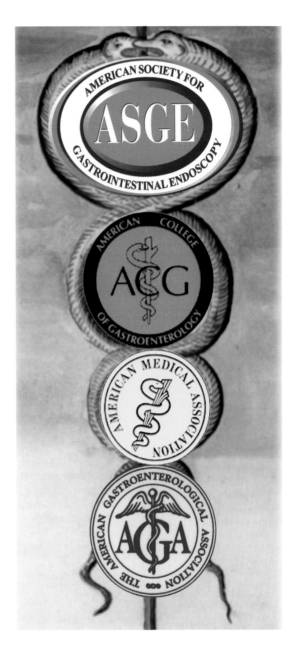

Much as the great city-states vied with each other for power in feudal Europe, so the territorial imperative of the various medical and gastrointestinal societies of the United States flourished as each sought to acquire eminent domain over the governance and boundaries of their respective fiefdoms. The meaning of the serpent emblem of Asclepius transmogrified as the Presidents of the various societies adopted the role of a *caduceator* bearing the eagle standards of its legion forwards to the political battles of Congress.

130

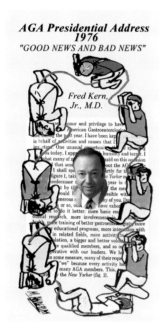

AGA Presidential Address 1976
"GOOD NEWS AND BAD NEWS"

Fred Kern,
Jr., M.D.

Fred Kern, a distinguished gastroenterologist and sage President of the American Gastroenterology Association in 1972, in his Presidential Address inveighed against the concept that the ASGE should "set standards" for endoscopy and publicly debated the wisdom of using "procedure numbers" as an arbitrator of competence and proficiency. His eloquent oral delivery and humorous cartoon (courtesy of Mrs. B. Kern.) paid immodest and satirical due to his vision of a world of endless endoscopy. Needless to say, not all accepted his position and the grim debate moved onward as a multi society committee was convened to formalize an understanding of the methodology whereby competency might be delineated.

ument acceptable to both groups be prepared. Although revised guidelines were developed and distributed to members of the ASGE for comment, a joint document issued by the ASGE and the AGA regarding training and practice was never produced.

Whilst the medical community in general accepted the concept of oversight, there were many who argued the right of the society to adopt this role. Since the AGA had already challenged the role of the society in setting standards, there existed a strong basis for disagreement. The situation was further exacerbated upon the decision of the Veteran's Administration (VA) System to adopt the guidelines proposed by the ASGE. Indeed the President of the AGA, Fred Kern, publicly chastised the leadership of the VA for accepting the ASGE guidelines and expressed concern that listing minimum numbers of procedures for satisfactory training would lead trainees to do unnecessary procedures to acquire the required number. He also raised the concern that measurement of skills by numbers was a flawed concept. As a result of this interchange the establishment of an intersociety committee to explore the issue of developing guidelines for training and practice in gastrointestinal endoscopy was suggested by the AGA. Members included representatives of the AGA, ASGE, the American Association for the Study of Liver Diseases, the American College of Gastroenterology, and the Society for Surgery of the Alimentary Tract. This group produced a unified statement of guidelines which stated that the recommended number of procedures for competency should be put in the appendix as a suggested number and that all indications that ASGE membership was a criteria for, or a judge of competency, be removed. The committee also declined to accept the issue of board certification in endoscopy and proposed review of this matter at an unspecified (sic) later date.

As a result of this tension between the AGA and the ASGE, further distance grew between the two organizations. This was compounded by the suggestion in 1975 by the AGA that endoscopy papers be included in their annual scientific session. Fortunately in 1976 John Morrissey established a more productive relationship with the AGA and a series of mutually supportive documents were thereafter produced by both groups. In 1977 the Gastroenterology Board published its *"Guidelines for Training of a Gastroenterologist"* and included for the first time guidelines for training in gastrointestinal endoscopy which subsequently became the basis for the development of special requirements for training in gastroenterology. Although similar to the ASGE guidelines, they differed specifically on the issue of the number of procedures required for competency by stating that the number would vary for each individual and should not be a set figure.

PUBLIC AWARENESS

In 1976 the National Commission for Digestive Diseases was created by an act of Congress. The mandate of this august group was to conduct a full study of the state of knowledge about digestive diseases, their social economic impact, facilities for research, diagnosis and prevention and make a long range plan for their control. The ASGE, and in particular John Morrissey, assumed a primary role in the deliberations of the Commission and contacted individual senators and representatives who had participated in the establishment of the commission. The President of the society, Bernard Schuman, testified before the commission providing articulate and cogent information regarding the aims and goals of the ASGE. As a result of its deliberations, the

Committee endorsed that standards of training for physicians be established in the society. They also recommended that the Federation of Digestive Disease Societies (FDDS) collaborate with the Joint Commission on Accreditation of Hospitals (JCAH) to establish the criteria for judging competency in endoscopy in the hospital setting. Despite the powerful support of the commission, the JCAH declined to adopt the guidelines proposed by the ASGE. The FDDS did, however, approve the guidelines of the society for training and it was therefore established that the five member societies (AASLD, ACG, AGA, SSAT, and ASGE) agreed to their relevance.

HISTORY AND EDUCATION

In 1972 the society appointed Martin Gordon of Yale to head a new History of Endoscopy Committee with a view to providing material for the Smithsonian Institute. The admirable efforts of Gordon culminated in the development of a unique collection of instruments that were initially housed at the Yale University Medical Library and displayed as a history of science exhibition. The interest generated by this important contribution led to the subsequent development of a traveling exhibit and a supporting film entitled "*Eyewitness to Gastroscopy-Revisited*", that became a significant adjunct to the activities of the society. Over a ten-year period this fascinating vignette of contemporary history entitled "*The Evolution of Gastroscopy — From the Magenkratzer to the Laser*" traveled to medical schools, museums, libraries and medical meetings throughout the United States. In 1978 an audiovisual library was established under the guidance of a subcommittee of the post graduate education committee. By the late 1970s a learning center that featured teaching materials and exhibits had been established as a regular part of the annual meeting.

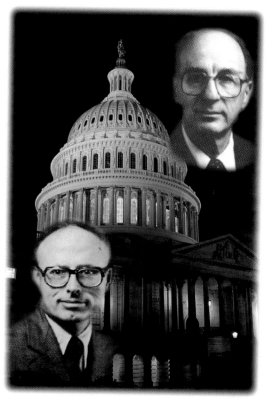

The visibility and impact of the ASGE in regard to its influence on the implementation of health policy was evident at the 1976 National Commission for Digestive Diseases created by an act of Congress. The position of the Society was provided by the testimony of two Presidents of the ASGE John Morissey (*top left*) and Bernard Schuman (*bottom left*), who espoused the Society's vision in the role of endoscopy in the health care delivery system of the nation.

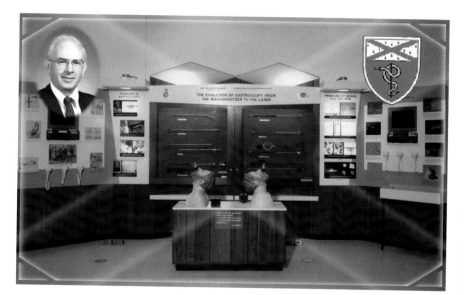

Martin Gordon (*left*) of Yale University School of Medicine in 1972 designed and assembled a historical collection of endoscopic instruments and documents that were initially housed at the Yale University School of Medicine library before becoming a popular travelling exhibit.

Administrative Mechanism

As the society grew in size, the administration needed refinement. In 1971 the secretary treasurer position was separated and a separate office for finance was established. This reflected the major increase in the responsibilities of the treasurer and as a result a professional relations and research institute represented by William Maloney was hired as executive director of the society and stabilized the administrative activities of the organization. In 1977 the company assumed the business management of the journal of *Gastrointestinal Endoscopy* and in so doing transformed the American Society for Gastrointestinal Endoscopy from its original modest beginnings into an international organization.

From Bulletin to Journal

William S Haubrich (*bottom left*) assumed the editorship of the journal in 1971 and by dint of scholarship and indefatigable energy was instrumental in establishing it as a major publication in the field of gastroenterology. Such was his success, that by the end of his tenure the undertaking had surpassed the limits of an individual and in 1979 the Williams and Wilkins publishing firm were hired to oversee the process.

The five years of the stewardship of Marvin and Palmer had initiated an intellectual and fiscal renaissance of the journal. Their able editorial leadership had not only resuscitated the *Bulletin*, but had enabled the attainment of financial viability and a maturation as a worthy and quotable scientific publication that was widely cited. In 1965 the name was reconfigured to embrace the broadening horizons of the field and the cognomen of *Gastrointestinal Endoscopy* replaced the former appellation of *Bulletin of....* Thus the humble 20 page *Bulletin* publication of 1961 had by 1971 amplified to a regular 50 to 60 page edition. Despite this substantial augmentation, the society maintained the subscription price for the four issues at $5 per year to ensure widespread access to topical material of such important educational significance. After a decade of fine service, Marvin retired as editor in 1971 and William S. Haubrich was appointed in his place. Such was his success that by 1979 the magnitude of the journal operation had become excessive for an individual and management was assumed by the publishing firm of Williams and Wilkins. Thus by the end of the decade both the journal and the society were recognized as leaders in world endoscopy and established as powerful voices in the arena of digestive disease.

In 1981 Bernard M. Schuman assumed editorship of the journal and under his direction new features and more color photography were added. In addition the size of the journal expanded and in 1984 the number of issues per year increased from four to six. This facilitated a rapid turnaround of original articles and by 1987 the journal published approximately 486 pages of text per year as compared with 170 in 1980. In 1989 Charles J. Lightdale became the editor and during his tenure the journal attained international educational status by publishing a number of important supplements, including: "*The Guidelines of the Society*", "*Endoscopic Ultrasonography*", "*Sedation and Monitoring*" and "*Therapy of Bleeding Ulcers*" in 1990. By 1990 the page number had risen to the unprecedented level of 658 pages per year in addition to 133 supplement pages. Such was the increase in the volume and quality of the material that in 1994 Lightdale, after 53 years of its publication, became the first editor to establish monthly publication of *Gastrointestinal Endoscopy*.

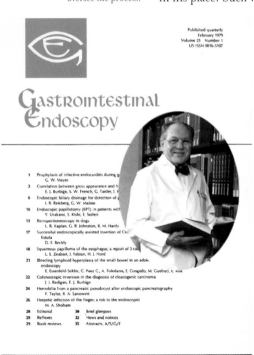

Published quarterly
February 1979
Volume 25 Number 1
US ISSN 0016-5107

Gastrointestinal Endoscopy

1 Prophylaxis of infective endocarditis during g
G. W. Meyer
3 Correlation between gross appearance and h
E. J. Burbige, S. W. French, G. Tarder, J. F
6 Endoscopic biliary drainage for detection of g
I. R. Reisberg, G. W. Mabee
10 Endoscopic papillotomy (EPT) in patients with
Y. Urakami, S. Kishi, E. Seifert
13 Retroperitoneoscopy in dogs
L. R. Kaplan, G. R. Johnston, R. M. Hardy
17 Successful endoscopically assisted insertion of Ce
fistula
D. E. Beckly
18 Squamous papilloma of the esophagus; a report of 3 cas
L. E. Zeabart, J. Fabian, H. J. Nord
21 Bleeding lymphoid hyperplasia of the small bowel in an adole
endoscopy
E. Essenfeld-Sektor, C. Paez C., A. Toledano, E. Congedo, M. Guelrud, E. Koa
22 Colonoscopic inversion in the diagnosis of cloacogenic carcinoma
J. J. Radigan, E. J. Burbige
24 Hemobilia from a pancreatic pseudocyst after endoscopic pancreatography
F. Taylor, R. A. Sanowski
26 Herpetic infection of the finger; a risk to the endoscopist
M. A. Shoham
28 Editorial   30   Brief glimpses
29 Reflexes   32   News and notices
29 Book reviews   35   Abstracts, A/S/G/E

American Society for Gastrointestinal Endoscopy

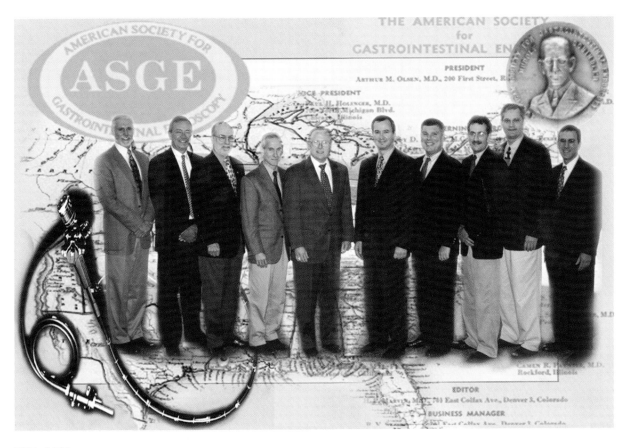

1981-1990

The advent of the 1980s brought with it recognition that the society had finally entered a phase of maturity. Jerome D. Waye in August of 1980 stated with confidence: "...the American Society for Gastrointestinal Endoscopy has matured. With
maturity the ASGE accepts its role as an equal but separate and individual member
of the medical and Gastroenterologic society." With the passage of time and secure
in the awareness of its successful evolution, the relationships between the ASGE, the
AGA, the ACG and the newly established Society of American Gastrointestinal
Endoscopic Surgeons (SAGES) flourished. A brief (once again) flirtation with the
possibility of an amalgamation with the AGA in 1982-3 considered the issue of a
possible merger but this failed to eventuate.

Overall the focus of the society during the 1980s was directed towards training,
education and accreditation. Diverse programs and committees were established to
undertake its complex and ever expanding role in the interface between gastroenterology and endoscopy. Thus individuals such as Steven E. Silvis, Joseph E. Geenen,
James Borland Jr., Walter J. Hogan, and Melvin Schapiro as the Chairmen of committees designated to provide guidance each played prominent roles in developing
different aspects of the society's activities. Issues of focus included the development of
an interface with the JCAH, assessing the role of conscious sedation, the development of self-assessment programs and the institution of endoscopic career development and research and education awards. An association was established with the
American Academy of Family Physicians (AAFP) and a Committee on Standards of
Training and Practice established in order to develop a uniform approach to teach-

The Governing Board of
the ASGE, 1999-2000.
Left to right: C.J. Gostout,
R.D. Baerg, H.J. Nord,
D.A. Lieberman, J.T.
Frakes (President),
M. Kimmey, MD,
L.S. Friedman,
D.J. Bjorkman,
R.H. Hawes, G.W. Falk.
Missing: D.L. Carr-Locke,
L.Y. Korman, R.A.
Kozarek,

ing. The extensive use of surveys by the society assured that the membership were in accord in maintaining its directions and priorities and facilitated maintenance of balance and perspective in a rapidly evolving medico-political environment.

At the end of the fifth decade of its existence the society had almost 5000 members and its annual dues had climbed to $140 per year. Its interests were diverse and involved the annual meeting, post graduate courses, the learning center, exhibits, investments, business matters and the establishment of an archive. Martin Gordon had laid the initial groundwork for the Archives committee and in 1980 Charles Lightdale assumed this responsibility. He was followed by Julian Katz in 1984, Lightdale in 1985, William Haubrich in 1986, and Bernard Schuman thereafter. Under Haubrich's guidance the documents and instrument collection were placed in a permanent home at the Cleveland (Ohio) Medical Library Association. The Presidential address of May 15, 1990 delivered by Michael V. Sivak Jr. appropriately concluded that the principles and direction of the ASGE have withstood the test of time!

1991 - 2000

As might be predicted the last decade of the millenium focussed the attention of the society on the rapidly developing interface between clinical and teaching requirements and the extraordinary advances of technology. Thus the sixth decade of the ASGE encompassed an explosion of novel endoscopic technology, including improved instruments, introduction of exotic therapeutic devices and other imaging modalities such as ultrasound. Such changes mandated a significant reconsideration of the Society's activities in consideration of technology assessment, research and education with a view to not only providing a degree of quality control for its membership but also ensuring that advances were appropriately deployed. Individuals of both experi-

Convocation of the past Presidents of the ASGE, Boston, 10.2.1999. *Left to right, back row*: Bernard. M. Schuman (1977-8), H. Juergen Nord (1998-9), H. Worth Boyce (1973-4), Bergein F. Overholt (1983-4), Francis J. Tedesco 1985-6), Michael V. Sivak, Jr. (1989-90), Bennett E. Roth (1994-5), Richard A. Kozarek (1997-8), James T. Frakes (1999-00), James L. Borland Jr. (1990-1), Emmett B. Keeffe (1995-96), David E. Fleischer (1993-94), Theodore R. Schrock (1986-7), Walter J. Hogan (1988-9) *Front row*: Jerome D. Waye (1980-1), Joseph E. Geenen (1982-3), Joel F. Panish (1979-80), William L. Maloney, Barbara B. Frank (1991-2), Melvin Schapiro (1984-5), John H. Bond (1992-3), Jeffrey L. Ponsky (1996-7) The background is the Allen Medical Library Building of the Cleveland Medical Library Association in Cleveland, Ohio. This historic edifice is home to the Dittrick Medical History Center that houses the venerable archives of the ASGE.

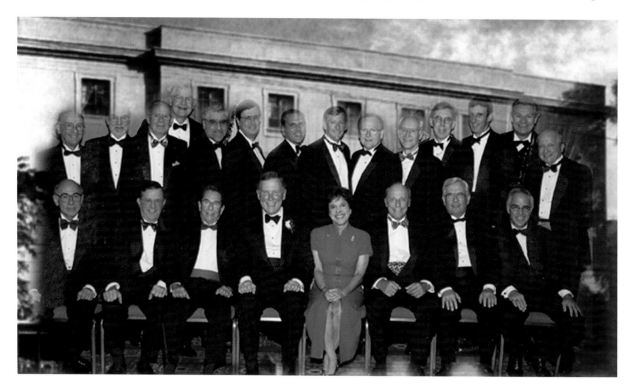

ence and clinical balance were entrusted with the task providing appropriate guidelines pertinent to establishing contemporary standards of training and practice consistent with the introduction of advanced and novel technology.

In addition to these exciting developments in the clinical and scientific arena the society was forced to marshal its energies in yet another direction as the somber reality of health care socio-economics began to cast a long shadow over its clinical endeavors. As a consequence of the machinations provided by increased legislative and regulatory activity coupled with the erosive influence of managed care organizations the economic viability of gastrointestinal endoscopy was exposed to serious constraint. Mindful of the necessity to maintain a viable position in the health care community the society responded with alacrity to such threats to its community and amplified its advocacy activity. Thus the Government Relations Committee was mandated to vigorously pursue the interests of the society and to further expand its reach was augmented by fission into two further committees, namely Health and Public Policy and Practice Management.

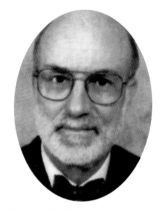

Juergen Nord, President of ASGE, 1998-9.

Notwithstanding the challenges provided by the current socio-economic milieu the society continued to focus strongly on its goals of education and research. In the attainment of such goals it was prescient in the adoption of both new approaches and novel teaching tools to enhance information transfer and learning. The number of teaching courses, tutorials, regional meetings and postgraduate courses were increased to accommodate the growing educational needs of its widespread caucus. To enhance and facilitate the intellectual and practical value of these scholarly exercises novel tools were acquired. Thus the introduction of visually effective and interactive digital video presentations, off site tele medicine seminars, hands-on tutorials at the Ethicon Institute and postgraduate courses not only became effective and popular learning tools but were further augmented by the development of the ASGE Internet web site. Mindful of the need to not only manage the present but prepare adequately for the future the Governing Board established a comprehensive blueprint to pursue enhanced fund raising for research. In this endeavor it was elected to actively petition the support of a number of organizations including the National Institutes of Health, the American Digestive Health Foundation as well as establish high profile public disease education and awareness campaigns. The latter goal was further amplified by internal societal focus on the development of a Foundation and the evolution of the Clinical Outcomes Research Initiative (CORI) project, in concert with proactive political representation in Washington. Indeed the positive health benefits that had accrued to many prominent politicians and even Presidents was cited as a compelling validation of the efficacy of the goals and achievements of the ASGE.

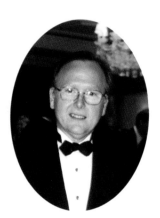

James Frakes, President of ASGE, 1999-2000.

As the sixth decade of the society neared its end and the century drew to a close, the ASGE membership had reached nearly 7,000 and the activities of its members had touched and benefited the lives of millions of Americans of all walks of life. The current President, James T. Frakes remarked "It is evident that endoscopy has traveled far and progressed greatly since the candle illuminated and mirrored tin tube days of Bozzini. Similarly, the ASGE as a society has both evolved and matured since the auspicious initial meeting in 1941 of 17 gastroenterologists in Schindler's apartment. It may be said that the society has not only preserved the light but nurtured and enhanced it for future generations of endoscopists." *Lux et Veritas*. Indeed the best that any society may hope for is that its light may bring truth and, in this case, health as well!

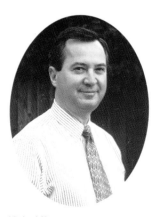

Michael Kimmey, President of ASGE, 2000-2001.

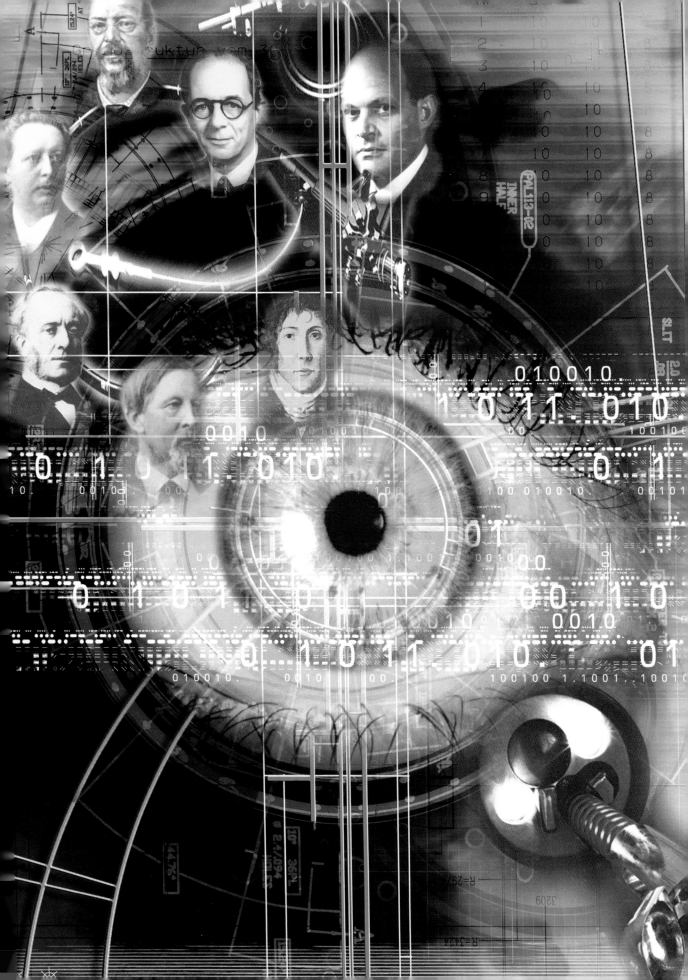

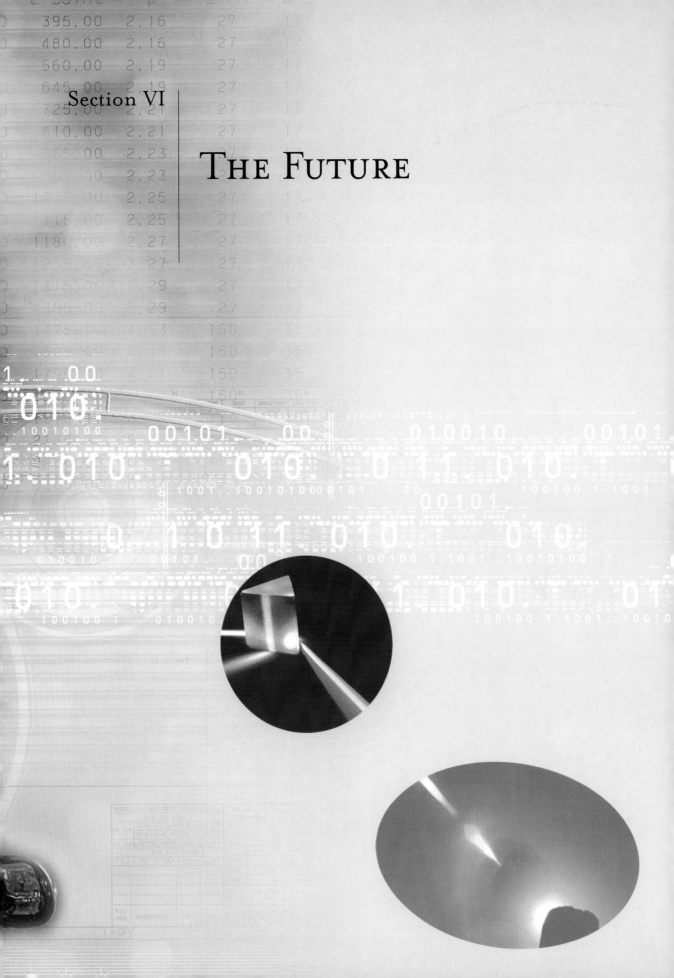

Section VI

THE FUTURE

THE FUTURE

While a review of the evolution of endoscopic instrumentation provides considerable insight into the past as well an understanding of the present, contemplation of the future is worthwhile. One may consider what pioneers such as Rosenheim, Mikulicz and Leiter thought in 1899 as they looked forward into the 20th century. They realized that adequate vision of the lumen was a priority, flexibility of the instrument a necessity, and patient safety and comfort an obligation. As we stand at the verge of the 21st century, the issues that confront us are not dissimilar and reflect considerations as to the requirements for the next century of endoscopy. Can we undertake the procedure without any patient discomfort at all? Will computers, robotics and different forms of visualization be implemented? Is it possible that instruments capable of determining cellular structure and biological behavior will supplant devices capable of a mere visual appreciation of mucosal structure? Will pattern recognition be supplanted by artificial neural circuitry and algorithmic formulation? Will the furthest reaches of the intestine be as amenable to examination as the proximal? What should be done to map the interior of the pancreas, bile ducts and liver? Will it be possible to not only enter these organs but to work within them? Lastly, will it be a possibility that endoscopists traditionally trained to function at an endo-luminal level lumen may extend their domain and address the bowel from the serosal aspect?

Dare we consider that the old disciplines of surgery and endoscopy be melded and that physicians involved in the care of gastrointestinal tract be the masters of all techniques rather than the purveyors of individual skills? Consideration should be given to the realization that the concept of a guild may well be overtaken by a matrix of modalities and that the disciplines of 1999 may become as archaic as the rigid endoscopes of 1899. The injunction of George Santyana (1863-1952): "Progress, far from consisting in change, depends on retentiveness... those who are not mindful of the past will be condemned to repeat it" should be heeded. Thus Isaac Newton, no stranger to the vagaries of light, in his discourse with Robert Hooke was mindful that future vision might be attained by reflection on the contributions of the giants of the past.

If the future of endoscopy is viewed in the most general terms we need to see further and see better. Once we have perceived there is a need to recognize the phenomenon, appreciate its structure and thereafter define it in pathological terms. At this juncture the ability to institute rational therapy becomes the crux of the matter. All such endeavor is fruitless if the information cannot be recorded, collated, shared and analyzed, since without evaluation the data becomes

Magnification endoscopy and contrast chromoscopy are areas that hold considerable promise in the amplification of pattern recognition and the early detection of lesions at the borderline of visual discrimination. Material courtesy of H. Mitooka (*inset*) of Kobe, Japan.

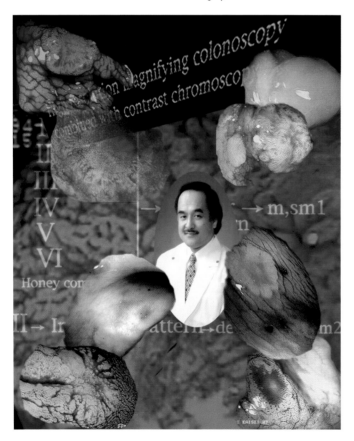

anecdotal and we remain in the "Old World" of apprenticeship and didactics. Indeed the path to management progress depends to a great deal on the accuracy, availability and assessment of current information.

Much as King Henry's first Portuguese "*discoberedos*" sought to see beyond Cape Bojador and Columbus sought to gain a New World, endoscopists have continually sought to round the next curve. It is likely that the concept of being tethered by a tube and limited by flexibility coefficients and length will be outmoded as transmission of imagery by waveform rather than solid circuitry supervenes. Under such circumstances, remote-control devices and self-propulsion technology may be predicted to replace the primitive contortions of manual-pulsion and torque maneuvers now in vogue. The technology currently utilized to direct and monitor information transmitted by remote units on the surface of Mars or the Moon is likely adaptable to terrestrial mucosa-oriented devices.

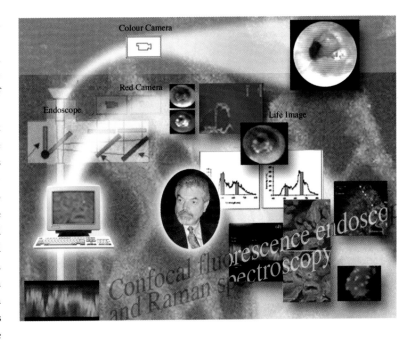

Once the area of interest is within range, the ability to identify and manage the problem is defined by the limits of spatial and white light resolution. Although magnification lenses and dye staining enhance pattern recognition, such modalities will be outmoded as the field of imagery moves beyond the boundaries imposed by visible wavelength light and macular acuity. Techniques including reflectance and light scattering spectroscopy will supplant optical fibers and charge-coupled devices in providing information in regard to mucosal and cellular events. The spectroscopic analysis of such signals using computer-generated analysis will enable the construction of 3-dimensional imagery of mucosal cellular architecture far beyond the simple visual discriminant index of the eye. Ultraviolet or laser generated light induced fluorescence endoscopy will utilize either endogenous or exogenous fluorophores to identify cells at a particular stage in their cell cycle. The use of a variety of laser probes to generate such excitation patterns at different wavelengths can be amplified by the administration of fluorescent sensitizers designed to augment recognition of specific cells or subcellular structures. This will further enhance detection of disease at a cellular as opposed to a macroscopic level. Similarly the use of pulsed-excitation sources and fast gated detectors can be used to further refine such signal acquisition and provide an even greater degree of sensitivity. Under such circumstances it is likely that the identification of specific constellations of cells in the process of transformation from the naïve-state can be defined. Resection or ablation prior to an autonomous growth pattern developing can then be preemptively undertaken. Indeed the entire concept of mucosal sampling for pathology based upon the assessment of histological biopsy material may radically alter as spectroscopy becomes adapted to determine and define the biological characteristics of proliferating tissue (dysplasia).

The application of optical coherence tomography, whereby light (energy) is delivered to the mucosa and the signal collected and quantified, will provide resolu-

The introduction of technology such as optical coherence tomography, Raman spectroscopy and fluorescence endoscopy will provide novel information equivalent to an "optical biopsy". Such devices possess the optical resolution capacity to not only indicate the biological status of the mucosa but also identify nuclear detail and delineate phenotype transformation. Material courtesy of N. Marcon, (*inset*), R.S. da Costa and B.C. Wilson, Toronto, Canada.

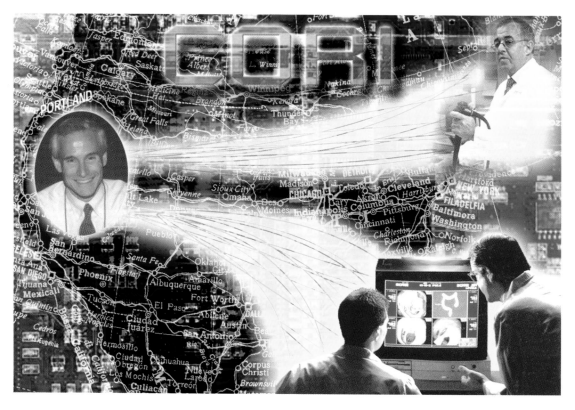

The interface of modern computer technology with endoscopic practice will amplify the ability of the discipline to assess imagery off site (tele medicine), guide procedures and facilitate teaching. The establishment of a sophisticated computer based system to network diverse endoscopic units throughout the United States has been implemented to establish a Clinical Outcomes Research Initiative (CORI) under the direction of D. Lieberman (*inset left*) of Portland, Oregon. A database of this power will provide real time information for analysis to determine and define indications, outcomes, management-policies and trend shifts in endoscopic care delivery.

tion of considerable detail. This technology will generate two-dimensional imagery that is ten fold greater than that available from endoscopic ultrasound. Image resolution as low as 2-4 μm is attainable and recognition of crypt architecture and even lymphoid aggregates is possible. Although the optical probes to deliver the light are currently available and pass through a standard biopsy channel, computers of considerable magnitude are required to assimilate the imagery and will predictably be developed.

Once a lesion is defined, the therapeutic aspects of endoscopy are the next challenge. Microscopic or cellular abnormalities may be ablated by lasers that have been rendered target specific by exogenous administration of cell specific dyes. Resection of areas of mucosa will utilize microscopic robotic controlled instrumentation. Such devices may be supported by the simultaneous application of trans peritoneal instruments delivered via laparoscopic ports, thus an area may be synchronously dealt with at both the mucosal and serosal level.

Bleeding should be controllable using endoscopic ultrasound directed microangiography or the direct application of clips, sutures or local vessel wall constrictive pharmacological agents. Laser probes capable of delivering targeted coagulation with micro capillary level accuracy will be supported by the post therapeutic introduction of biological shields that will be anchored for sufficient time to provide a "coffer dam" within which healing of the mucosal lesion can occur. The development of similar devices constructed from a variety of biologically compatible polymers can function either as stents or as endo-liners to cover mucosal tears or perforations. Adherent liners of this type may also be impregnated with coagulation agents, cytotoxics or growth factors and used to provide local delivery of pharmacotherapeutic agents.

If the medium is the message and the light the truth, then data acquisition and retrieval as epitomized by the application of computer technology and the development of artificial intelligence and neural networks is the mantra of the future. Such technology may safely be predicted to play an even greater role in a future endoscopic world. Similarly the use of electronic image transmission and tele medicine technology will facilitate real time off site evaluation and transfer care beyond the limited boundaries of dedicated medical environments. The likelihood of the availability of robotic and self-propelled miniaturized devices will further amplify such developments and swallowing a "video pill" may in the future render the manual dexterity of the endoscopic maestro as quixotic as the techniques of a Caravaggio or Rembrandt in an age of DVD imagery.

One may say with little fear of contradiction that at this time the view beyond the lens is clear, exciting and infinite. As the peripatetic sage Nivri Nildom noted, "the pursuit of vision and light has indeed opened the doors of truth to the lumen of knowledge. Yeah verily, the macula has seen the mucosa and beyond".

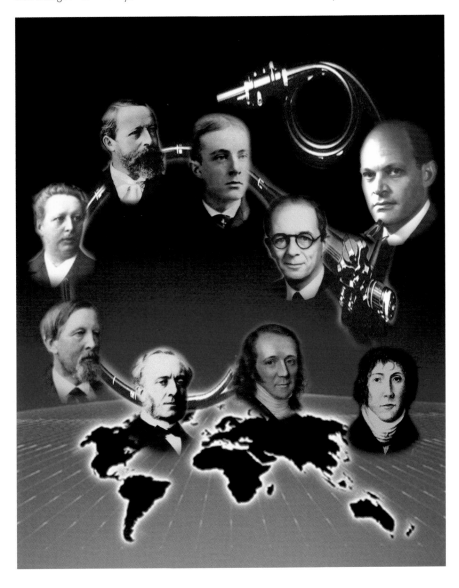

The Pioneers of Endoscopy.
From 5 o'clock clockwise:
Philip Bozzini (1773-1809), Pierre Segalas (1792-1875), Antonin Desormeaux (1815-1881), Adolf Kussmaul (1822-1902), Max Nitze (1848-1906), Johann Mikulicz (1850-1905), Chevalier Jackson (1865-1958), Rudolf Schindler (1888-1968), Basil Hirschowitz (1925-). Each a physician of perspicuity and persistence, undaunted by failure and frustration, they labored mightily against the vicissitudes of their times to safely pass the dark lumen in their search for knowledge and cure.

References

Section I

1. Modlin I.M. *From Prout to the Proton Pump.* 1995. Konstanz, Schnetztor-Verlag GmbH. Konstanz

2. Garrison Fielding H. *Contributions to the History of Medicine.* 1966. New York, Hafner Publishing Company, Inc.

3. Morton's Medical Bibliography. 5th Edition. 1991, Ed. J.M. Norman.

4. Kussmaul A. *Memoires of an old Physician.* 1981. New Delhi, Amerind publishing Co. Pvt. LTD.

5. Bast T.H. *The life & time of Adolf Kussmaul.* 1926. New York, Paul B. Hoeber Inc.

6. Friedenwald J. and Morrison S. *The history of the development of the stomach tube with some notes on the duodenal tube.* Bull. Hist. Med. 4, 425-454. 1936

Section II

1. Reuter H.J. *Philipp Bozzini and endoscopy in the 19th century.* 1988. Stuttgart, Max Nitze Museum.

2. Reuter M.A, Reuter H.J., Engel R.M. *History of Endoscopy.* Stuttgart. 1999.

3. Bozzini P. *Lichtleiter, eine Erfindung zur Anschauung innerer Theile und Krankheiten nebst der Abbildung.* Hufelands neues Journal der pract Heilkunde 17, 107-124. 1806.

4. Ringleb O. *Zur Erinnerung an Philipp Bozzini.* Zeit Urol 17, 321-330. 1923.

5. Lesky E. *Die Wiener Experimente mit dem Lichtleiter Bozzini.* Clio. Med 5, 327-350. 1970

6. Hausmann H. *Philipp Bozzini.* Z.Urol.u.Nephrol. 77, 729-734. 1984.

6. Segalas M. *Description of an instrument for inspecting the urethra and bladder.* Lancet 11, 603-604. 1826.

7. Hayes I. and Fisher J.D. *1827 Endoscope.* Philadelphia J. Med. Phys. Sci 14, 409. 1827.

8. Desormeaux A.J. *De l'endoscope, instrument propre a eclairer certaines cavites intensely de l'economie.* Comptes rendues de l' Academie des Sciences 40, 692-693. 1855.

9. Cruise F.R. *The utility of the endoscope as an aid in the diagnosis and treatment of disease.* Dublin Q J Med Sci. 39, 329-363. 1965.

11. Nitze M. *Eine neue Beobachtungs- und Untersuchungsmethode für Harnröhre, Harnblase und Rektum.* Wien Med Wschr 24, 650. 1879.

12. Leiter J. *Elektro-endoskopische Instrumente.* 1880. Wien, W. Braumüller & Sohn.

13. Murphy Leonard J.T. *The History of Urology.* Desnos E. *L'Histoire de l'Urologie.* 1999. Springfield, Ill., USA, Charles C. Thomas.

14. Huizinga O. *On esophagoscopy and sword swallowing.* Ann. Otol. 78, 32-39. 1969

15. Mikulicz J. *Ueber Gastroskopie und Oesophagoskopie.* Wien Med Wschr 33, 705. 1883

16. Rosenheim Th. *Ueber Gastroskopie.* Berl Klin Wschr 33, 275-278. 1896

17. Einhorn Max. *Diseases of the Stomach.* Third revised Edition. 1943. New York, William Wood and Co.

18. Baird J.L. *An improved method for and means for producing optical images.* British patent 285, 738. 1928.

19. Hopkins H. and Kapany N.S. *A flexible fiberscope using a static scanning.* Nature 173, 39-41. 1954.

20. Hecht J. *City of Light: The Story of Fiber Optics* (Sloan Technology Series). Oxford Univ Press. 1999.

21. Jackson Ch. *Gastroscopy: Report of Additional Cases.* J Amer. Med. Assoc. 49, 1425-1428. 1907.

22. Kelling G. *Ueber Oesophagoskopie, Gastroskopie und Kölioskopie.* Munch.Med Wochenschr 52, 21-23. 1902.

23. Schindler R. *Gastroscopy in thirty cases of gastric neoplasm.* Arch Intern Med 32, 635-646. 1923.

24. Schindler R. *Gastroscopy with a flexible gastroscope.* Am J Dig Dis Nutr. 2, 656. 1935.

Section III

1. Sternberg W. *Fortschritte und Rückschritte in der Gastroskopie.* Acta Chir Scand 55, 563. 1923.

2. Sauerbruch F. *Gastroskopie mit tödlichen Ausgang.* Zentralblatt für Chirurgie 38, 2071-2072. 1924.

3. Chamberlin D.T. *Description of a new gastroscope.* Gastroenterology 12, 209-211. 1948.

4. Schindler R. *Gastroscopy with a flexible gastroscope.* Am. J Dig Dis Nutr. 2, 656. 1935.

5. Schindler R. *Gastroscopy-the endoscopic study of gastric pathology.* 1937. Chicago, University of Chicago Press.

6. Schindler R. *Lehrbuch und Atlas der Gastroskopie.* 1923. Munich, JF Lehmans.

7. Schindler R. *On the importance of the gastroscope in the diagnosis of gastric diseases in the army.* Brit. Med J 17, 243-247. 1940.

8. Schindler R. and Ortmayer M. *Classification of chronic gastritis with special reference to the gastroscopic method.* Arch Intern Med 57, 959-978. 1936

9. Edmonson J.M. *History of Instruments for Gastrointestinal Endoscopy,* Gastrointestinal Endoscopy 37, 2, S27-56. 1991

10. Davis, A.B. *Rudolf Schindler's role in the development of gastroscopy.* Bull Hist.Med. 46, 150-170 (1972).

11. Gordon, M.E. & Kirsner, J.B. *Rudolf Schindler, pioneer endoscopist. Glimpses of the man and his work.* Gastroenterology 77, 354-361 (1979).

12. Kirsner, J.B. *American gastroscopy—yesterday and today.* Gastrointest. Endosc. 37, 643-648 (1991).

13. Schindler R. *George Wolf.* Am J Dig Dis., 817-818. 1938.

14. Hett J.H. and Curtiss L.E. *Fiber Optics Duodenoscope and Ureteroscope.* J. Opt. Soc. Am. 51, 581-582. 1961.

15. Weiss S. *A New Gastroscope for Visualization and Photography.* Am. Med. 15, 547-548. 1930.

16. Palmer W.L. *The stomach and the military service.* JAMA, 119, 11551159. 1942

17. Janeway H.H. *Esophagoscopy and gastroscopy.* Surgery Gynecol. Obstet. 13, 245-252. 1911.

18. Herrick F.C. *Profuse recurrent gastric hemorrhage, with report of cases and description of an instrument for viewing the gastric interior.* Cleveland Med J 10, 969-976. 1911.

19. Hemmeter J.C. *Diseases of the Stomach.* 1902. Philadelphia, P. Blakiston's Son & Co.

20. Benedict E.B. *Examination of the stomach by means of a flexible Gastroscope: a preliminary report.* New Engl. J. Med. 210, 669-674. 1934.

21. Hufford A.R. *Flexi-rigid, optical esophagoscope.* Gastroenterology. 12: 779-781. 1949

22. Segal H.L. and Watson J.S. Jr. *Color photography through the flexible gastroscope.* Gastroenterology 10, 575-585. 1948

Section IV

1. Hirschowitz B.I., Curtiss L.E., Peters C.W., and Pollard H.M. *Demonstration of a new gastroscope, the "fiberscope".* Gastroenterology 35, 50-53. 1958

2. Hirschowitz B.I. *Endoscopic examination of the stomach and duodenal cap with the fiberscope.* Lancet 1: 1074-78. 1961

3. Cohen N.N., Hughes R.W. Jr., Manfredo H.E. *Experience with 1000 fibergastroscopic examinations of the stomach.* Am. J Dig. Dis. 11:943-950.1966

4. LoPresti P.A., Hilmi A.M. *Clinical experience with a new foroblique fiber optic esophagoscope.* Amer. J Dig. Dis. 9, 690-697. 1964

5. McCune W.S., Shorb P.E., Moscovitz H. *Endoscopic cannulation of the ampulla of Vater: a preliminary report.* Gastrointest. Endosc. 34, 278-280. 1988

6. Demling L., Koch H., Classen M., Belohlavek D., Schaffner O., Schwamberger K., Stolte M. *Endoscopic papillotomy and removal of gall-stones: animal experiments and first clinical results.* Dtsch Med Wochenschr .99(45):2255-7 1974

7. McCune, W.S. *ERCP at thirty years: an interview with Dr. William S. McCune (1909-1998).* Gastrointest. Endosc. 48, 643-644 1998.

8. McCune, W.S. *ERCP—the first twenty years.* Gastrointest. Endosc. 34, 277-278 1988.

9. Oi I., Takemoto T. and Kondo T. *Fiberduodenoscope: direct observation of the papilla of Vater: a preliminary report.* Endoscopy 3. 101-103. 1970

10. Zimmon D.S., Falkenstein D.B., Kessler R.E. *Endoscopic papillotomy for choledocholithiasis.* N. Engl. J. Med. 293(23):1181-2 1975

11. Kelly H.A. *A new method of examination and treatment of diseases of the rectum and sigmoid flexure.* Ann. Surg. 21, 468-478. 1895.

12. Turell R. *Fiber optic coloscope and sigmoidoscope. Preliminary report.* Amer. J Surg. 105. 133. 1963.

13. Provenzale L., Camerada P. and Revignas A. *La coloscopia totale trans-anale mediante una metodica originale.* Rass Med Sarda. 69. 149. 1966

14. Overholt, B.F. *Clinical experience with the fibersigmoidoscope.* Gastrointest. Endosc. 15, 27.1968.

15. Overholt, B.F. *Flexible fiberoptic sigmoidoscopes.* South Western Med. J. 63: 787-789, 1969.

16. Wolff W. I. and Shinya H.A. *A new approach to colonic polyps.* Ann. Surg. 178. 367-376. 1973

17. Kelling G. *Ueber Oesophagoskopie, Gastroskopie und Kölioskopie.* Munch.Med Wochenschr 52, 21-23. 1902.

18. Bernheim B.M. *Organoscopy.* Ann Surg 53, 764-767. 1911.

19. Kalk H. *Erfahrungen mit der Laparoskopie.* Zeit Klin Med III, 303-348. 1929.

20. Jacobaeus H.C. *Ueber die Möglichkeit die Zystoskopie bei der Untersuchung seröser Höhlungen anzuwenden.* Munch.Med Wochenschr 57, 2090-2093. 1910.

21. Ruddock J.C. *Peritoneoscopy.* Surgery Gynecol. Obstet. 65, 623-639. 1937.

22. Benedict E.B. *Peritoneoscopy.* New Engl J Med 218, 713-719. 1938.

23. Nadeau O.E. and Kampmeier O.F. *Endoscopy of the abdomen; Abdominoscopy.* Surgery, Gynecol. Obstet. 41, 259-271. 1925.

24. Ponsky J.L., Gauderer M.W. *Percutaneous endoscopic gastrostomy: a nonoperative technique for feeding gastrostomy.* Gastrointest. Endosc. 27 (1):9-11. 1981